Dear Reader,

Healthy hands enable you to interact with the world: they touch, feel, manipulate, emote, and communicate. Their strength allows you to grip, pinch, and carry. Their coordination provides the ability to engage in fine, intricate tasks. But when the exquisite architecture of the bones, ligaments, muscles, tendons, and nerves is damaged through injury or wear, all of those capabilities you normally take for granted can become painful, challenging, or even impossible.

In this report, we highlight the major conditions that can affect your hands and help you understand what options exist to remedy these problems. We detail disorders that can affect the joints, including different types of arthritis, and describe ways to reduce the associated pain and disability using assistive devices, medications, and surgery. We cover carpal tunnel syndrome and other nerve issues, including how treatment can help you reclaim your sensory function and get a better night's sleep. This report also highlights tendon problems and other ailments specific to the hands, such as Dupuytren's disease and trigger finger. Finally, we show you ways to protect your hands from overuse and injury so they may continue to work for you—all day, every day.

This report draws on the expertise of its two medical editors—one of us a hand surgeon, the other a hand therapist. Over our combined 41 years of practice, the two of us have worked together to treat thousands of patients. During that time, we have come to appreciate the importance of teamwork and collaboration in taking care of issues involving the hands. Some can be managed well without surgery, while others benefit from surgical repair and hand therapy to safely restore the fullest function possible.

We hope that this report will give you a new appreciation for the intricate architecture of hands and that it will help you to keep yours as healthy as possible.

Sincerely,

Brandon E. Earp, M.D.
Medical Editor

Gayle B. Lang, M.S., O.T.R./L, C.H.T.
Medical Editor

The editors would like to thank Barry P. Simmons, M.D., and Joanne P. Bosch, M.S.P.T., C.H.T., who created the original version of this report. Their expertise, knowledge, and wisdom continue to permeate this, the updated edition.

The healthy hand

It's hard to imagine getting through a day without using your hands. Beyond their countless practical functions, like opening doors, preparing food, and tying shoelaces, we use these complex structures in many other ways, to both convey and perceive information.

People who can't speak or hear use their hands to converse through sign language. But even people with normal hearing use their hands to communicate—by throwing them in the air in frustration, by applauding, or by touching someone's shoulder. You may clench your hands in anger or clasp them together in prayer. Your hands can even offer clues to your personality (consider a warm, firm handshake).

People who can't see use their hands to read, thanks to the exquisite sensitivity of the fingertips. Although your sense of touch extends throughout your body, your hands are the main organ you use to gather tactile information about your environment.

Hand structure and physiology

Because the hands perform many functions, it's no wonder they have a complicated design (see Figure 1, page 3). Sadly, complexity can also lead to trouble.

Bones. Each of your hands has 27 bones. Together, the 54 bones in your two hands make up a quarter of the total bones in your body. However, their number and proximity means that if one thing goes wrong, it can also affect nearby parts of the hand and wrist.

Muscles, tendons, and ligaments. To control movement, each hand has 34 muscles, which are found in the palm and forearm. About a quarter of the brain's motor cortex (the part that controls all movement in the body) is devoted to the muscles of the hands. But surprisingly, there are no muscles in the fingers—only ligaments and tendons.

Tendons in the hand connect muscles in the forearm to bones of the fingers and thumb. The job of flexing and extending the fingers (or wrists, elbows, and so forth) falls to tendons. When a muscle contracts, it pulls on the tendon, which then pulls on the bone and moves it. Flexor tendons, on the palm side of the hand, help you bend, or flex, your fingers, while extensor tendons, on the back of the hand, help you

The remarkable human thumb

You may have heard that an opposable thumb is one key anatomical difference that distinguishes humans from animals. Actually, many animals—including chimpanzees, koalas, and even opossums—have opposable thumbs, which means they can oppose, or touch, the thumb to the index finger. But humans have a unique ability to also oppose the thumb to the other fingers, thanks to flexible joints in those digits. It's this ability that allows you to strongly grip and grasp objects. About 40% of the hand's function is attributed to the thumb.

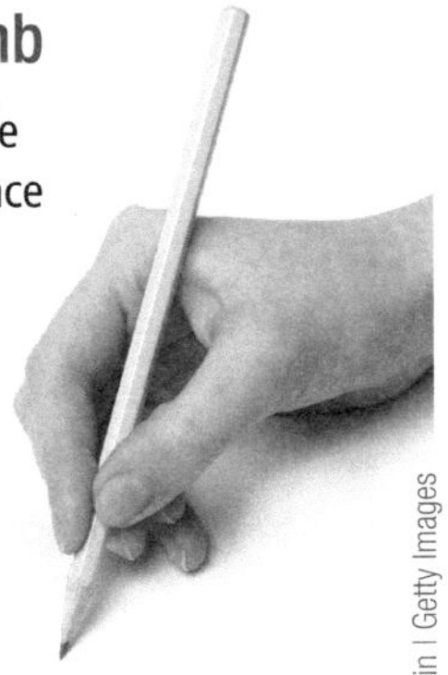

Opposable thumbs that can touch all the other fingers give human beings their dexterity.

Other thumb facts

- The word thumb comes from the Latin *tumere*, meaning "to swell"—a nod to its short, thick form.
- Because of the shape of the joint at the base of the thumb, it is able to move in a larger circular pattern than the other fingers.
- The slight hollow on the dorsal (top) side of the wrist at the base of the thumb is known as the anatomical snuff box, so named because snuff (powdered tobacco) could be put there and inhaled.
- Also referred to as the first finger or pollix, the thumb has three bones (two in the thumb itself and one that connects it to the wrist). That's one fewer than the other fingers.
- People who are born without a complete thumb or who lose one in an accident can undergo pollicization—the surgical creation of a thumb from a finger, usually the index finger. Another option for replacing a lost thumb is a toe-to-thumb transfer.

straighten them. An entire chapter of this report is devoted to tendon troubles.

While tendons attach muscle to bone, ligaments bind bone to bone, holding the bones together and keeping them in proper alignment. The ligaments on either side of your finger joints prevent excessive side-to-side deviation, while the ligaments that stretch across your palm keep your fingers from bending too far back.

Both tendons and ligaments consist of tough connective tissue fibers made of collagen, the protein that gives them the strength and flexibility to perform their distinct functions. Because these fibrous tissues have little blood supply, however, tendon and ligament injuries heal slowly.

Tendons in the hand are largely covered by protective sheaths that resemble deflated balloons. The inner lining, or synovium, produces a clear, slippery fluid resembling egg white, called synovial fluid. (In fact, the word comes from the Greek prefix *syn-* and the

Figure 1: Inside the hand

Under the skin, the hand's 27 bones and 34 muscles work in synchrony to perform a range of movements, from a powerful hammer blow to a gentle caress.

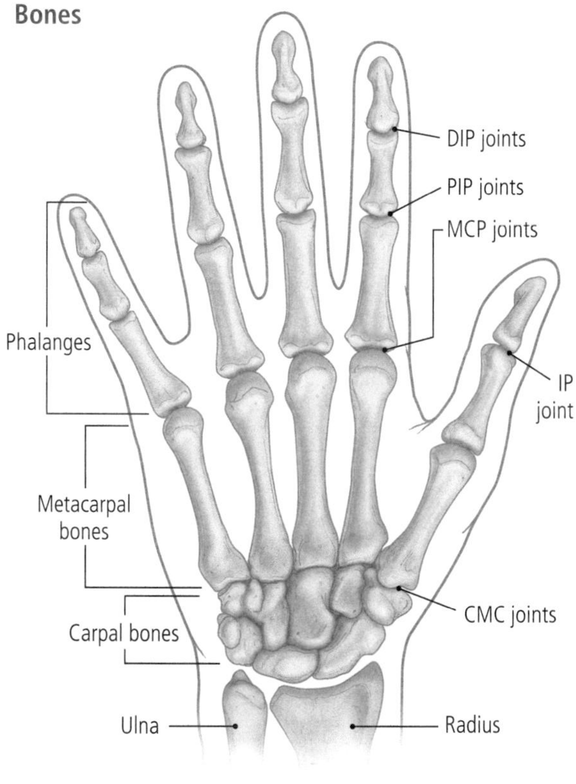

The main bones of the hand are the metacarpals, which connect to the finger bones, or phalanges. The knuckle joints that connect these bones are the metacarpophalangeal (MCP) joints. Each finger has three phalanges, and the thumb has two. The middle joint of the finger is the proximal interphalangeal (PIP) joint. The joint near the end of the finger is the distal interphalangeal (DIP) joint. Instead of DIP and PIP joints, the thumb has one interphalangeal (IP) joint. The major bones of the wrist are the carpals, which connect to the ends of the larger forearm bones, the ulna and radius. The carpals connect to the metacarpals at the carpometacarpal (CMC) joints.

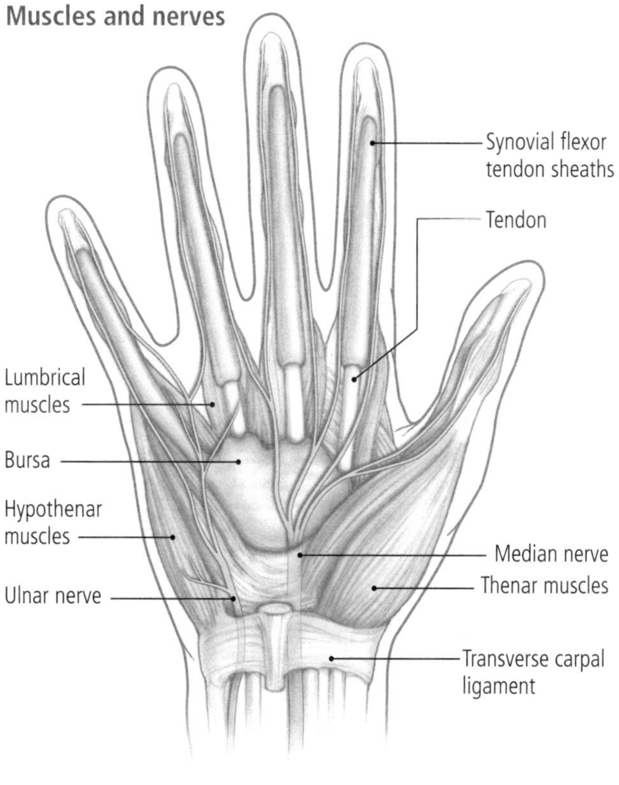

The small but powerful muscles of the hand are located entirely in the palm and forearm. The fingers have no muscles. Fingers are controlled by tendons attached to the muscles of the hand that help to bend and straighten them. Two major nerves are the median nerve (which provides sensation to the thumb, index, and middle fingers and the inner half of the ring finger) and the ulnar nerve (which provides sensation to the pinky and the outer half of the ring finger). The bursa helps cushion the hand.

Latin word *ovum* and means "with egg.") The joints, too, are lined with synovium and filled with synovial fluid. This vital substance lubricates tendons and joints, providing frictionless movement of the fingers. It also supplies nutrients to nearby bones and cartilage.

Cartilage. This tough and somewhat elastic tissue cushions joints and provides a smooth, slick surface for movement. When it degrades, this leads to osteoarthritis, one of the leading problems of the hand.

Nerves. Three major nerves (the radial, median, and ulnar) serve the hand. The median nerve, which passes through the wrist, is noteworthy because pressure on this nerve causes carpal tunnel syndrome.

The nerves in your hands also gather crucial information about the world around you and enable you to react swiftly. For example, why do most people instantly withdraw their hand when their fingers touch a hot object? The credit goes to a complex sensory system, including closely packed nerve endings in the skin, connective tissue, and joints of the hands that detect pressure, light touch, vibration, joint position, heat, and pain. This sensory system relays information through the peripheral nerves and spine to the somatosensory cortex of the brain, which processes the information and forwards the message to the motor cortex, so the body can respond. If nerves are cut or compressed, the system is disrupted, diminishing the ability to distinguish between touch, pain, and changes in pressure and temperature and to tell where the sensations are coming from.

The nerves are also essential for things like gripping and pinching, which depend on hand and wrist position, forearm and hand muscles, and the positioning of fingers. Grips are divided into several types, depending on the position of your thumb and fingers: power grip (with fingers flexed toward your palm, as when grasping a suitcase handle); cylindrical grip (wrapping thumb and fingers around an object but not touching each other, as when holding a drinking glass); and fist grip (wrapping thumb and fingers around an object, as when holding a hammer or squash racket). Pinches are divided into two major types: three-point pinch (with fingers on one side of an object and thumb on the other, as when holding a pencil); and lateral pinch (with thumb against the side of the index finger, as when holding and using a

How a certified hand therapist can help

A certified hand therapist is either an occupational therapist or a physical therapist who has specialized education and training in rehabilitation of the hand. This specialist evaluates your hand's range of motion and strength, as well as any pain, swelling, or physical limitations caused by your condition. He or she then applies a wide range of therapies to help you regain normal use of your hand. Common conditions that may warrant seeing a hand therapist include arthritis, tendinitis, carpal tunnel syndrome, or trigger finger.

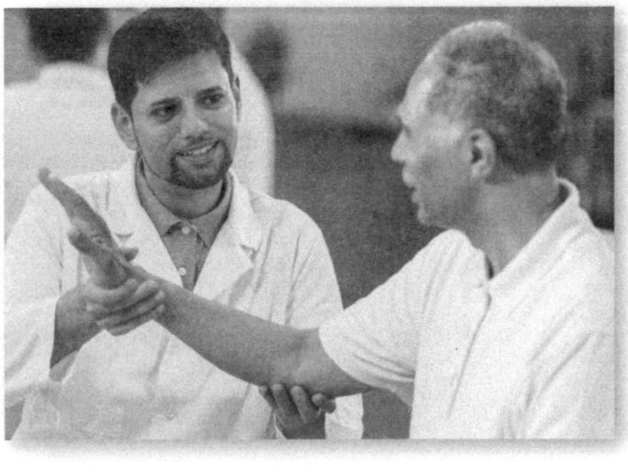

A hand therapist's tool kit includes such varied treatments as massage, heat or ice applications, and ultrasound to warm and increase blood flow to muscles and joints. The therapist can also teach you how to relieve pain and stiffness at home by dipping your hands in warm paraffin wax melted in an electric appliance that maintains a safe temperature. After the wax hardens, you wrap the treated area in a plastic sheet and blanket to retain the heat.

Do not be surprised if a therapist also gives you a set of hand exercises to increase your strength and range of motion (see "Exercises for the hands," page 43). He or she may also fabricate a custom-made splint to provide rest or support for a particular part of your hand (see "Splints," page 24).

Beyond relieving immediate pain, hand therapists can help you prevent future damage to your hands by showing you how to use ergonomic tools that relieve stress on your hands, and how to set up your work space and position your body to protect your joints. They can also show you how to modify your movements and pace your activity to speed recovery.

To find a hand therapist, ask for a recommendation from the orthopedist or primary care physician who diagnosed your hand problem, or contact the Hand Therapy Certification Commission (see "Resources," page 50). Note that insurance coverage of hand therapy services varies; check your plan for details.

key). Grip strength is used as an indicator of health in the elderly, with a weaker grip strength one sign of frailty.

Professionals who treat hand problems

Your primary care practitioner can diagnose and treat certain hand conditions. But in many cases, he or she may refer you to a doctor such as a rheumatologist, who specializes in arthritis and related conditions, or a general orthopedist, who specializes in muscle, tendon, bone, and joint disorders. Orthopedists are also trained in treating the forearms, elbows, and shoulders (known collectively as the upper extremities).

Hand surgeons are orthopedic, plastic, or general surgeons who have additional training in surgery of the hand. They diagnose and treat problems of the hands, wrists, and upper extremities using both surgical and nonsurgical techniques.

Occupational and physical therapists also treat hand problems. People with hand conditions may be referred to a hand therapist before seeing other physician specialists. Hand therapists teach exercises, help with proper body movement and posture, and give advice on ergonomics, with the goal of increasing strength and mobility and preventing recurring injuries. These specialists also recommend treatments, splints, and devices that make it easier to carry out the tasks of daily living, both at home and at work. A certified hand therapist is an occupational or physical therapist with at least three years of experience who specializes in rehabilitating people with hand conditions and passes a national exam on hand therapy (see "How a certified hand therapist can help," page 4). Some even specialize in treating people from particular professions, such as musicians or athletes. In this report, the term "therapist" refers to any of these professionals.

Did you know?

About 10% of people are left-handed. Perhaps because they're in the minority, the Latin word for left, *sinister*, also came to mean unlucky or inauspicious. Popular notions abounded that lefties were more prone to accidents or illnesses. Studies have failed to uphold those assertions. However, living left-handed in a right-handed world can be awkward. Items as common as scissors, clothing clasps, and door handles—all designed for righties—conspire to make everyday life more difficult. That said, the ranks of high achievers are filled with notable lefties, including Marie Curie, Babe Ruth, and five of the past nine U.S. presidents.

Arthritis of the hand

Joint inflammation, or arthritis, is the leading cause of disability among Americans, causing stiffness, swelling, pain, and loss of motion and function. There are more than 100 kinds of arthritis, including osteoarthritis and rheumatoid arthritis. Arthritis can affect any joint in the body, but it is especially visible when it affects the hands.

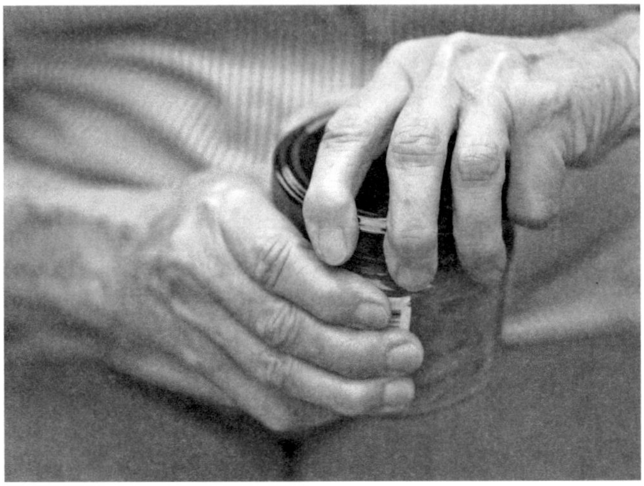

© bloodstone | Getty Images

Stiff, achy joints can make it hard to open a jar. However, a hand therapist can work with you to find ergonomic tools and assistive devices that help modify tasks.

Osteoarthritis

The most common of all joint diseases, osteoarthritis affects cartilage, the tissue that cushions the ends of your bones within a joint. Normally, cartilage provides a smooth, gliding surface so the joints can move easily. In osteoarthritis, the cartilage thins and loses its elasticity. As the cartilage breaks down, the underlying bone may form a bony growth called a spur, or osteophyte. Fluid-filled cysts may form in the bone or in soft tissues near the joint (see "Finger cysts," below). The synovial membrane lining the joints becomes inflamed, triggering the release of proteins that may damage the cartilage further.

More than 32.5 million Americans have osteoarthritis. In addition to the hands, osteoarthritis most commonly affects the knees, hips, feet, and spine. The incidence rises with age, with most cases occurring in people older than 50. Heredity seems to play a role in a person's susceptibility to arthritis, particularly for osteoarthritis in the hands. Muscle weakness and a history of joint injuries caused by sports or accidents may also make a person more prone to a type of osteoarthritis known as post-traumatic arthritis. Ordinary, repetitive activities such as typing or playing a musical instrument may worsen arthritis symptoms, but they do not cause osteoarthritis of the hands.

Finger cysts

Mucous cysts are clear or flesh-colored nodules that form on the fingers under the skin near the DIP joints. They occur most commonly in middle-aged or older women with osteoarthritis. These cysts often don't cause any symptoms, but sometimes are tender and painful and may limit your finger mobility, leading to stiffness and deformity. They rarely go away on their own and may drain spontaneously and become infected, requiring prolonged antibiotic treatment. More stubborn cysts may require a hand surgeon, who will open the joint and remove the cyst as well as any associated bone growth or spur (osteophyte).

Diagnosing osteoarthritis

To diagnose any type of arthritis, your doctor may order blood tests to rule out other possible causes of your symptoms. He or she will ask specific questions

Symptoms of osteoarthritis

- ✔ Pain in the morning, which gradually recedes but returns at the end of the day
- ✔ Pain that is alleviated by resting the affected joint
- ✔ Stiffness in the affected joint

about your symptoms, such as when they first started and how they affect your life. Details of your personal and family medical history may also be relevant.

Your doctor will take x-rays of the affected joints, which can reveal evidence of bone spurs and narrowing of the joint space between the bones. This narrowing signifies cartilage breakdown within the joint. Most people older than 60 have some signs of arthritis on an x-ray, but only about one-third have symptoms. There is often a big difference between the severity of osteoarthritis seen on an x-ray and how much pain and disability a person feels; some people with severe arthritis on x-ray don't have many symptoms, while others with mild arthritis on x-ray can have a lot of pain.

Certain joints of the hands are especially susceptible to osteoarthritis:

The distal interphalangeal (DIP) joint—the last joint before the nail on each finger (see Figure 1, page 3)—is the most common site for osteoarthritis of the hands. These joints sometimes develop fibrous, bony nodules called Heberden's nodes.

The basal or first carpometacarpal (CMC) joint—located at the base of the thumb, where the thumb and wrist come together—is the second most common joint to develop osteoarthritis of the hands. Past injuries to this joint, such as a fracture or sprain, may increase the odds of getting arthritis in this joint.

The proximal interphalangeal (PIP) joint—the middle joint of each finger—can also develop osteoarthritis, causing the fingers to stiffen and swell. Fibrous and bony nodules, known as Bouchard's nodes, may develop in these joints.

The metacarpophalangeal (MCP) joints—where the fingers join the rest of the hand—are sometimes affected by osteoarthritis as well. These knuckle joints act as hinges between the long bones in the hand and the smaller bones in the fingers. Swelling of these joints is common in people with rheumatoid arthritis. Injuries or other diseases, such as gout or psoriasis, can also cause problems in these joints.

Treating arthritic hands

Managing pain and improving function are the key goals in treating osteoarthritis. The best approach is usually a combination of therapies, which can include splinting, joint protection, heat or cold therapy, exercise, medication, alternative remedies, and, in some cases, surgery.

Splinting. The first line of action for treating arthritis hand pain is splinting to immobilize the joint. This allows the joint to rest so the initial pain can subside. Splints can be used to support the painful joint during the day or at night.

Joint protection. If you have osteoarthritis, it's important to learn to recognize your body's signals to stop or slow down. A hand therapist can help you with this. To prevent pain caused by overexertion, take time to rest, and pace yourself by taking frequent breaks. Using specialized ergonomic tools and assistive devices can also make a big difference (see "Getting a grip: Handy gadgets and advice," page 47). Modifying tasks to make them less stressful allows you to continue to do the things you need or want to do while alleviating the symptoms of arthritis.

Heat or cold therapy. You can often soothe painful joints without medications. Soaking your hands in warm water can ease pain and stiffness and make it easier to do recommended hand exercises. Other

Does knuckle cracking cause arthritis?

Cracking your knuckles may provoke an annoyed grimace from those around you, but it probably won't raise your risk for arthritis. That's the conclusion of several studies that compared rates of hand arthritis among habitual knuckle-crackers and people who didn't crack their knuckles.

The "pop" of a cracked knuckle is caused by bubbles bursting in the synovial fluid. The bubbles pop when you pull the bones apart, either by stretching the fingers or bending them backward, creating negative pressure. One study's authors compared the sudden, vibratory energy produced during knuckle cracking to "the forces responsible for the destruction of hydraulic blades and ship propellers."

Even if knuckle cracking doesn't cause arthritis, there's still good reason to let go of the habit. Chronic knuckle-crackers were more likely to have swollen hands and reduced grip strength. And there are at least two published reports of injuries suffered while people were trying to crack their knuckles.

times, usually after exercise or exertion, cold therapy may work better. You can place a bag of ice or frozen vegetables wrapped in a towel on the joint or use a freezer gel pack, available at drugstores. Check with a doctor or therapist to find out whether heat or cold is the best treatment for you.

Exercise. Exercise helps people with osteoarthritis in many ways: by increasing flexibility and strength, decreasing pain, and improving mood and general fitness. Therapeutic exercises, especially range-of-motion exercises for the thumb and wrist, help keep hand joints working as well as possible (see "Exercises for the hands," page 43). Gentle, pain-free strengthening may be appropriate once localized swelling and pain have subsided. Activities to improve dexterity may help counter weakness in small muscles of the hands. Consult a hand therapist for specific exercises for your hand problem, since doing the wrong type of exercise for your particular condition may make the problem worse.

Topical pain relievers. There are a number of medications for arthritis, starting with topical pain relievers (see Table 1, below). One over-the-counter gel, diclofenac (Voltaren Arthritis Pain Gel), offers modest relief for hand arthritis. Other over-the-counter gels and creams haven't been studied as thoroughly, but some people find them helpful for treating mild to moderate pain. Topical products containing CBD (cannabidiol, a non-psychoactive component of marijuana) are widely available, but there is only weak evidence of their effectiveness based on animal studies, and the amount of the active ingredient and purity of the formula is not consistent from one brand to the next—sometimes even within a brand. Topical medications may be a good choice for people with gastrointestinal conditions, since they're absorbed directly through the skin and have a more localized effect.

Oral medications. For more severe pain, oral medications are typically more effective. Those that

Table 1: Topical pain relievers

Topical pain relievers work best on joints close to the skin surface, such as those in the hands. One of these, diclofenac, is available over the counter as a gel or by prescription as a patch; both forms relieve mild to moderate joint pain and inflammation. The others, also available over the counter, are moderately effective for mild pain. None, however, will alter the course of arthritis. Do not use these on broken or irritated skin or in combination with a heating pad or bandage.

GENERIC NAME (brand name)	ACTIVE INGREDIENT	HOW IT WORKS	SIDE EFFECTS	COMMENTS
capsaicin (Capzasin, Zostrix, others)	Derived from cayenne peppers	Depletes substance P, which is believed to send pain messages to the brain	Temporary burning or stinging at the application site, which usually disappears within a few weeks of continuous use	Wash your hands thoroughly after use. Avoid contact with the eyes.
counterirritants (ArthriCare, Eucalyptamint, Icy Hot, Therapeutic Mineral Ice, others)	Include pungent oils derived from mint, wintergreen, eucalyptus, and other plants	Stimulate or irritate nerve endings to distract the brain's awareness of pain	Skin redness and irritation at application site	Many of these products have strong odors.
diclofenac (Flector Patch, Voltaren Arthritis Pain Gel, others)	A nonsteroidal anti-inflammatory drug (NSAID)	Inhibits hormone-like substances (prostaglandins) that contribute to pain and inflammation		Do not use with oral NSAIDs. Long-term users of either product should receive periodic blood tests to monitor liver function. All NSAIDs slightly increase the risk of heart attack and stroke, but levels that reach the bloodstream are far lower with topical application.
salicylates (Aspercreme, Bengay, Flexall, Mobisyl, Sportscreme, others)	A type of NSAID derived from willow tree bark	Same as for both diclofenac and counterirritants		Do not use if you are allergic to aspirin or are taking blood thinners.

are in the class known as nonsteroidal anti-inflammatory drugs (NSAIDs), such as the over-the-counter pain relievers ibuprofen (Advil, Motrin) and naproxen (Aleve), curb inflammation in addition to pain (see Table 2, below). A drug used for rheumatoid arthritis, hydroxychloroquine (Plaquenil; see Table 3, page 13), has been tested but found to be ineffective in reducing symptoms of hand osteoarthritis.

Injections. For short-term relief, corticosteroids, known informally as steroids, can be injected directly into a joint to relieve pain. Be aware, however, that excessive injections increase the destruction of bone and cartilage over time.

Alternative or complementary therapies. These span a range of options, including acupuncture and dietary supplements. (See "Alternative and complementary treatments for arthritis," page 10, for more information.)

Surgery. This option usually is recommended only after other treatments have failed. Several surgical procedures are used for osteoarthritis, each one focused on treating the symptoms at a particular joint. One common surgery is the removal of cysts and osteophytes at the DIP joint. Another is surgery for arthritis at the base of the thumb. People with severe osteoarthritis may be candidates for joint fusion or joint replacement (see the Special Section, page 18).

Rheumatoid arthritis

Rheumatoid arthritis is much less common than osteoarthritis. Still, it affects about more than 1.3 million Americans, about 75% of them women. Certain genes may make people more likely to have the disease, which can run in families.

A chronic inflammatory condition, rheumatoid arthritis most commonly strikes the small joints of the wrist, hands, and feet. However, it can also attack the joints in the neck, shoulders, elbows, hips, knees, and ankles. Misshapen fingers that make many everyday tasks difficult are one telltale sign of advanced disease. Rheumatoid arthritis usually affects both sides of the body in a fairly symmetrical fashion. Affected joints often swell, feel warm and tender, and are especially stiff and painful when you wake up or after you rest.

The disease is widely considered to be an auto-

Symptoms of rheumatoid arthritis

- ✔ Swelling, warmth, and stiffness in the affected joints, especially in the morning or after rest
- ✔ Usually affects joints on both sides of the body
- ✔ In some cases, also fatigue, loss of appetite and energy, fever, or anemia

Table 2: Over-the-counter oral pain relievers

All of these medications except acetaminophen are NSAIDs. Avoid NSAIDs if you have gastrointestinal problems, and take them with food, milk, or an antacid to minimize stomach irritation. NSAIDs other than aspirin slightly increase the risk of heart attacks and strokes.

GENERIC NAME (brand name)	USE	SIDE EFFECTS	COMMENTS
acetaminophen (Tylenol, others)	Relieves pain	Nausea, vomiting, diarrhea, jaundice, rash, tiredness, weakness; less likely to cause gastric bleeding than other pain relievers	Drinking large amounts of alcohol during long-term therapy with acetaminophen may cause liver damage. Risk of liver damage is also increased if you exceed 3,000 mg per day. Acetaminophen is found in many medications, so keep track of your total intake. Kidney damage also possible with long-term use.
aspirin (Bayer, Ecotrin, others)	Reduces inflammation and relieves pain	Stomach pain, bleeding, ulcers	High doses may cause ringing in the ears. Before using, let your doctor know if you are on blood thinners or have liver or kidney problems.
ibuprofen* (Advil, Motrin, others)			Stronger and generally longer-lasting than aspirin.
naproxen* (Aleve)			Longer-lasting than ibuprofen.

**Ibuprofen and naproxen are available in higher doses by prescription only. Naproxen is also sold by prescription in combination with a medication to suppress stomach acid (either lansoprazole or esomeprazole), under the brand names Prevacid NapraPAC 500 and Vimovo.*

immune disorder, meaning the body's immune system mistakenly attacks its own organs or tissues. In rheumatoid arthritis, the immune system attacks the synovium (joint lining), which then releases enzymes that destroy nearby cartilage. This causes redness, pain, and swelling. Eventually, the joints become enlarged, hindering normal movement. Your fingers may swell and appear sausage-shaped, and you may develop a soft, lumpy mass over the back of your hand. You may hear a creaking sound (called crepitus) when you move your fingers.

Over time, the ligaments and tendons that hold bones in place stretch and weaken, causing your bones to become misaligned. The MCP joints are often affected. Your fingers may shift toward the pinky side of your hand, away from the thumb, a problem known as ulnar deviation or ulnar drift. The pain and deformity can be quite debilitating. It may become difficult to hold a cup, tool, or eating utensil. Other daily tasks such as combing your hair and buttoning your shirt can be challenging. (See "Getting a grip: Handy gadgets and advice," page 47, for tips on coping with these limitations.)

Inflammation from rheumatoid arthritis can cause the tendons to swell and sometimes rupture, resulting in an inability to bend or straighten the fingers. These tendon injuries can create characteristic deformities. One condition of this type is called a boutonniere deformity, from the French word for buttonhole, so named because it involves a small tendon tear that resembles a buttonhole. Another is a swan-neck deformity, in which the middle joint of the finger (the PIP joint) hyperextends and the joint at the end of the finger (the DIP joint) droops (see Figures 2 and 3, both on page 11).

Diagnosing rheumatoid arthritis

In addition to a medical history and physical exam, doctors use both imaging and lab

Alternative and complementary treatments for arthritis

Many people with chronic, painful conditions like arthritis who don't get complete relief from conventional therapies turn to alternative treatments. As with any therapy, some people find that certain treatments work well for them, while others find little or no benefit. Talk with your physician to decide which approaches might work best for you, and consult a licensed, certified practitioner for specific treatment and guidance. *The discussion below does not constitute an endorsement of any of these treatments.*

Acupuncture and acupressure. These ancient Chinese therapies have become popular for treating pain-related conditions, and some studies have shown acupuncture to be effective for some forms of pain. A 2013 analysis also indicates that the therapy can be useful in the treatment of gout. In a 2019 randomized study, people with rheumatoid arthritis of the hands who underwent acupuncture gained better grip strength and reduced pain and swelling, while those on a waiting list or undergoing a fake acupuncture treatment did not improve.

Diet. Several studies indicate that there is a connection between diet and the systemic inflammation that characterizes rheumatoid arthritis. A diet emphasizing fruits and vegetables, olive oil, fish, and whole grains—similar to the Mediterranean eating pattern—may reduce inflammation.

Dietary supplements. A number of vitamins, minerals, and other substances are sold as remedies for arthritis. Because these products are classified as dietary supplements, they are not scrutinized for effectiveness and purity by the FDA. The following supplements have been tested for various forms of arthritis within the past decade:

- **Boswellia serrate (Indian frankincense).** In a meta-analysis combining two studies, patients who took the supplement for 90 days reported slightly less pain and increased function compared with individuals who took a placebo.
- **Curcumin (turmeric).** In a monthlong trial, supplements containing curcumin—a naturally occurring anti-inflammatory compound in the spice turmeric—were as effective as ibuprofen in treating knee osteoarthritis, with fewer gastrointestinal side effects.
- **Glucosamine and chondroitin sulfate.** Limited research has been conducted on glucosamine and chondroitin sulfate—two components of cartilage that are sold as supplements—for osteoarthritis of the hand. In a 2020 comparison, people who took glucosamine sulfate in addition to standard therapy (hand exercises and pain relievers) had less pain and better hand function three and six months later than those who received standard therapy alone. In the United States, glucosamine is usually sold in combination with chondroitin sulfate.

tests to diagnose rheumatoid arthritis. No single lab test can confirm whether a person has rheumatoid arthritis, but several blood tests can help clarify the diagnosis. For example, about 80% of people with rheumatoid arthritis have an antibody known as rheumatoid factor in their blood, although they may not have it early on. Another blood test is for C-reactive protein (CRP), which is a sign of inflammation. Additional lab testing for gout, Lyme disease, and other ailments may be used to distinguish rheumatoid arthritis from these other causes of swollen, painful joints.

X-rays can reveal swelling of soft tissues, bone loss around the joints, and bone damage (called erosions) near the joints. More sophisticated imaging tests such as magnetic resonance imaging (MRI) can detect early inflammation, even before it's visible on an x-ray, such as synovitis (inflammation of the lining of a joint) and tenosynovitis (inflammation of the protective sheath around a tendon).

Figure 2: Two common finger problems from rheumatoid arthritis

When inflammation damages tendons and ligaments that normally keep a joint straight, the fingers can become deformed.

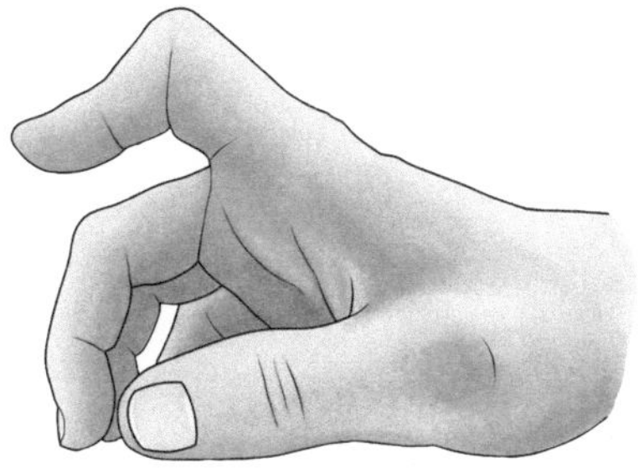

Boutonniere deformity results from damage to tendons that straighten the middle joint of the finger.

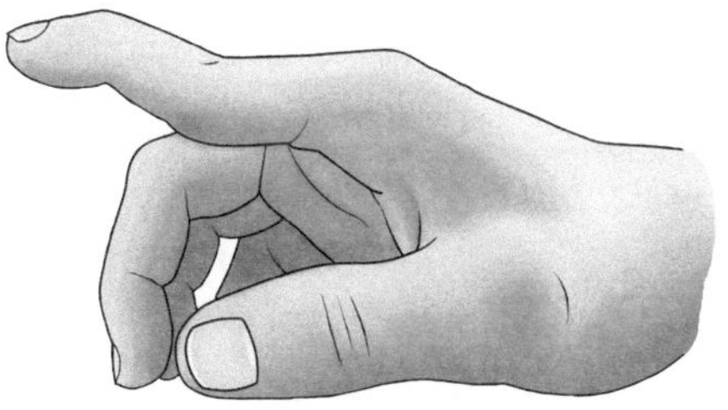

Swan-neck deformity occurs when inflammation stretches ligaments that keep fingers in proper alignment.

Treating rheumatoid arthritis

As with osteoarthritis, doctors recommend oral and topical painkillers (see Table 1, page 8, and Table 2, page 9), and, in some cases, oral corticosteroids to help manage pain and swelling. But decades of research show that early treatment with powerful drugs known as disease-modifying antirheumatic drugs (DMARDs) can reduce inflammation, reduce or prevent joint damage, and lessen the chance of long-term disability from rheumatoid arthritis for some people. As a result, most people with rheumatoid arthritis take a DMARD, usually methotrexate (Trexall, others), often as the initial medication prescribed following diagnosis.

For people with more serious disease, other options are drugs that work by inhibiting specific components of the immune system to block inflam-

Figure 3: Hands with rheumatoid arthritis in many joints

These photos and x-rays come from two patients and show some of the many hand problems that can occur in rheumatoid arthritis. The pointers highlight just a few of them.

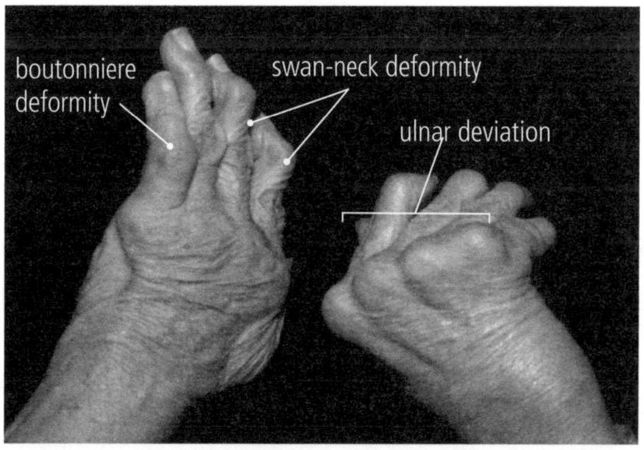

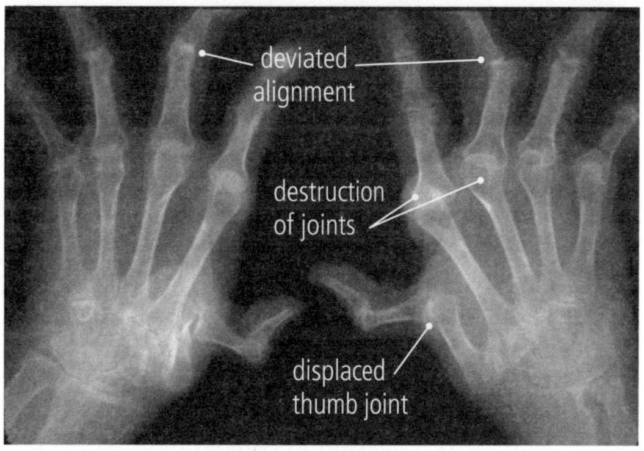

Images reprinted with permission, Barry P. Simmons, M.D.

mation and joint damage. These drugs fall into two groups:

- Biological response modifiers (also called biologics) are created through genetic engineering of proteins from human cells. They are given via injection or intravenous infusion and inhibit inflammation-causing components of the immune system, such as tumor necrosis factor (TNF).
- Targeted DMARDs inhibit enzymes called kinases at points along a specific pathway by which the immune system signals an attack on the joints. Targeted DMARDs are not created using genetic engineering. They are taken orally.

Both biological response modifiers and targeted DMARDs can be prescribed in addition to a DMARD such as methotrexate (see Table 3, page 13, for more details).

Because DMARDs have proven so successful in managing the symptoms of rheumatoid arthritis and lessening joint destruction, hand surgeons have seen a reduction in the number of people who need surgery. But for those whose symptoms become debilitating despite medication, surgery is an option. Surgery for rheumatoid arthritis strives to reduce pain and improve function, and can also improve the appearance of your hands.

Soft tissue removal (particularly procedures known as synovectomy and tenosynovectomy) involves removing diseased tissue from the tendons and joints. The surgeon may also reposition some tendons and release others to stop the fingers from drifting toward the little finger. Although synovectomy can decrease pain and swelling and slow joint destruction, the condition may recur. However, use of DMARDs dramatically decreases recurrence.

In rare instances, surgeons replace wrist joints (and in some cases, MCP and PIP joints) destroyed by rheumatoid arthritis (see the Special Section, "Joint reconstruction for arthritic hands," page 18). In some cases, it is preferable to fuse two bones together surgically to stabilize and alleviate the pain in a joint.

Physical or occupational therapy for rheumatoid arthritis of the hands is similar to treatment for osteoarthritis and includes splinting, joint protection, pacing (planning of activities and rest breaks), ergonomics, and gentle exercise. These therapies may be key to managing your symptoms and regaining function. It's important to seek medical advice early because it may help you detect when the condition is getting worse so you can begin treatment to prevent deformities.

Other types of arthritis that affect the hands

Several other, less common types of arthritis, including gout and pseudogout, can cause debilitating hand symptoms. In addition, conditions such as lupus, scleroderma, and psoriatic arthritis may cause arthritic symptoms that involve the hands.

Gout

A small percentage of arthritis cases are related to gout, a condition caused by deposits of tiny, needle-like crystals that form when the body either makes too much uric acid or excretes too little of it. Uric acid forms from the breakdown of purine, a substance found in protein-rich foods. The symptoms of gout resemble those of rheumatoid arthritis (joint pain, tenderness, warmth, and redness), but gout tends to affect only one joint at a time, and it may begin suddenly—often in the middle of the night. Pain may be quite severe and tends to resolve within a few days. Gout is most common in the big toe joint (a condition known as podagra). However, it often affects other joints in the feet, ankles, and hands, as well as elsewhere in the body.

Anyone can get gout, but it's most common in men older than 40. In women, it is most likely to develop after menopause. Gout occurs in about 1% to 4% of people over all, but as many as 6% to 7% of older men. Being overweight and drinking alcohol increase

Continued on page 14

Symptoms of gout

- ✔ Jolts of pain in the affected joint
- ✔ Possible inflammation of the joint
- ✔ Increase in symptoms after eating certain foods

Table 3: Medications for inflammatory arthritis

These medications are prescribed for people with rheumatoid arthritis and related types of inflammatory arthritis, such as psoriatic arthritis.

GENERIC NAME (BRAND NAME)	SIDE EFFECTS/COMMENTS
▶ Oral corticosteroids These medications reduce pain by suppressing inflammation. Abruptly stopping oral steroids after taking them for more than 10 to 14 days can cause a life-threatening condition called Addisonian crisis. For this reason, the drugs must be taken exactly as prescribed.	
methylprednisone (Medrol) prednisone (Deltasone, Orasone, others)	Side effects include fluid retention, weight gain, facial hair growth, easy bruising, loss of calcium from bones, cataracts, and sleeplessness, among others. Side effects are related to dosage and length of therapy. If a low dose is taken for a week or less, side effects are rare. If therapy continues for months or years, side effects are more noticeable, even at low doses.
▶ Disease-modifying antirheumatic drugs (DMARDs) These powerful drugs are prescribed early to relieve pain and swelling, limit joint damage, and alter the course of the disease.	
hydroxychloroquine (Plaquenil) leflunomide (Arava) methotrexate (Trexall, others) sulfasalazine (Azulfidine)	Can take weeks or months to work. Side effects vary with each medication and include increased risk for infection, hair loss, stomach upset, rash, and kidney or liver damage. Methotrexate can suppress the immune system and may cause birth defects. Leflunomide may also cause birth defects. All DMARDs require close supervision and monitoring by a physician.
▶ Targeted DMARDs Most of these drugs inhibit kinases, enzymes involved in inflammation and joint damage. They are used for moderate to severe rheumatoid arthritis or other inflammatory arthritis in people who do not respond to methotrexate. Apremilast inhibits a different enzyme (PDE4) and is approved for use in psoriatic arthritis.	
apremilast (Otezla) baricitinib (Olumiant) tofacitinib (Xeljanz, Xeljanz XR) upadacitinib (Rinvoq)	Pills taken once or twice daily. Reduce inflammation. Common side effects include diarrhea, headache, runny or stuffy nose, sore throat, nausea, fever, shingles, and upper respiratory infections. Suppress the immune system. Serious side effects of kinase inhibitors include infections, cancers, and blood clots. All kinase inhibitors require close medical supervision and monitoring of lab results. Apremilast may cause severe diarrhea, nausea, or vomiting, new or worsening depression, and weight loss.
▶ Biological response modifiers These drugs, also known as biologics, are created from genetically engineered proteins derived from human cells. Given by injection or intravenous infusion, they inhibit specific components of the immune system, such as tumor necrosis factor (TNF), helping to suppress inflammation and slow the progression of rheumatoid arthritis.	
Anti-TNF compounds: • adalimumab (Humira) • certolizumab (Cimzia) • etanercept (Enbrel) • golimumab (Simponi) • infliximab (Remicade)	Side effects vary depending on the medication and include an increased risk for infections, from colds and sinus infections to more serious diseases such as tuberculosis.
Other biological response modifiers: • abatacept (Orencia) • anakinra (Kineret) • guselkumab (Tremfya) • ixekizumab (Taltz) • rituximab (Rituxan) • sarilumab (Kevzara) • secukinumab (Cosentix) • tocilizumab (Actemra) • ustekinumab (Stelara)	Side effects vary but may include nausea, diarrhea, heartburn, muscle or back pain, tiredness, weakness, numbness in the hands or feet, stomach area pain. Tocilizumab may cause serious infections, diverticulitis, severe allergic reactions, and increases in blood lipids.

Continued from page 12
your risk for gout. Research suggests that men who eat generous amounts of red meat and seafood are more prone to gout. Those who eat more dairy products are less likely to be affected.

To diagnose gout, doctors measure uric acid levels in the blood and take a sample of fluid from the joint to look for uric acid crystals under a microscope. But uric acid levels aren't always elevated during an attack, and many people with high levels never develop gout. Some people develop lumpy deposits made of sodium urate (called tophi) around the joints.

At the first sign of a gout attack, your doctor may prescribe colchicine (Colcrys, Mitigare) to reduce pain and inflammation in your joints. This drug prevents white blood cells from accumulating around uric acid crystals. Your doctor may also recommend NSAIDs or corticosteroids.

Some people with gout take drugs to lower uric acid levels in their blood. These include probenecid (Benemid, Probalan) to increase urinary excretion of uric acid, and allopurinol (Aloprim, Lopurin, Zyloprim), febuxostat (Uloric), and pegloticase (Krystexxa) to reduce the body's production of uric acid. Lesinurad (Zurampic), which has a different mechanism for increasing uric acid excretion, is used in combination with allopurinol or febuxostat.

Pseudogout

As its name suggests, pseudogout is similar to gout, except that the crystals in the joints are made of calcium pyrophosphate dihydrate. The condition is often referred to as calcium pyrophosphate deposition disease, abbreviated as CPDD. Like gout, pseudogout causes redness, heat, and swelling in one or more joints, including those in the wrists and knees. The body attacks the crystals, which can cause swelling that may damage nearby cartilage.

About 3% of people in their 60s develop pseudogout, although not all of them will have attacks. No one knows why some people develop these crystals, but they may result from an abnormality in the cartilage cells or connective tissue. Genes may also have an influence, and people with certain other medical conditions, including hypercalcemia (excessive calcium in the blood), hypothyroidism (low activity of the thyroid gland), and hemochromatosis (excess iron in the blood), are more prone to the problem.

Samples of joint fluid can help doctors diagnose pseudogout, and x-rays may reveal the calcium deposits in the joint. Drug treatments for pseudogout include NSAIDs and corticosteroids. Sometimes removing joint fluid through a needle improves the condition without additional treatment.

Lupus

An autoimmune disease related to rheumatoid arthritis, lupus can affect various parts of the body, especially the skin, blood, and kidneys, as well as the joints—including multiple joints in the hand and wrist. Also called systemic lupus erythematosus (SLE), the disease affects women about eight to 10 times as often as men, most commonly between the ages of 18 and 45. Lupus-related arthritis in the hands tends to cause less swelling and joint damage than rheumatoid arthritis, but it may affect similar joints and feel the same.

Some people with lupus develop hand deformities similar to those seen in rheumatoid arthritis, such as ulnar deviation at the MCP joints and swan-neck deformities (see Figure 3, page 11). Lupus can be hard to diagnose because there isn't a specific set of symptoms that occurs in everyone who has the disease. The workup may include several different blood tests, as well as urine analysis, chest x-rays, and heart tests.

Medications for lupus include over-the-counter

Symptoms of pseudogout

- ✔ Jolts of pain in the affected joint
- ✔ Redness, warmth, and swelling in the affected joint

Symptoms of lupus

- ✔ Swollen, achy joints
- ✔ Fever (100° F or higher)
- ✔ Prolonged or extreme fatigue
- ✔ Rashes

painkillers (see Table 2, page 9) and some drugs used to treat rheumatoid arthritis, such as methotrexate and hydroxychloroquine, an antimalaria drug (see Table 3, page 13). For people whose lupus fails to respond to these medications, the biologic drug belimumab (Benlysta), delivered by intravenous infusion or injected just under the skin, is an option.

Scleroderma

This autoimmune disease commonly affects the hands and fingers. Derived from the Greek words meaning "hard skin," scleroderma is also a connective tissue disease, meaning it affects major substances in the skin, tendons, and bones. It can be either localized (affecting limited areas of the skin, muscles, and bones) or systemic (causing more widespread skin changes and sometimes damaging the lungs, heart, and kidneys). It is quite rare, with only about 20 new cases diagnosed per million people each year, mostly in women.

People with scleroderma often have some or all of the symptoms that doctors refer to as CREST, which stands for the following:

- **Calcinosis:** the formation of calcium deposits (visible on x-rays) in connective tissues, usually in the fingertips, face, and trunk, and on the skin above the elbows and knees. Painful ulcers may form where the deposits break through the skin.
- **Raynaud's syndrome:** a condition that occurs when small blood vessels in the hands or feet contract in response to cold (see "Cold hands: Is it Raynaud's syndrome?" on page 16).
- **Esophageal dysfunction:** a condition caused by muscle problems in the esophagus (the tube that connects the throat and stomach), making swallowing difficult and sometimes causing chronic heartburn.
- **Sclerodactyly:** thick, tight skin on the fingers, stemming from too much connective tissue within skin layers. Bending or straightening the fingers becomes difficult, and the skin may become shiny, dark, and hairless. The fingertips become tapered and may develop ulcers.
- **Telangiectasias:** small, painless red spots on the hands and face caused by the swelling of tiny blood vessels.

Symptoms of scleroderma

- ✔ Hard, thickened skin that appears shiny and may lose hair
- ✔ Swollen, puffy fingers and toes with poor blood flow and extreme sensitivity to cold
- ✔ Ulcers or sores on fingertips
- ✔ In some cases, digestive, heart, lung, or kidney problems

Doctors also rely on blood tests, and possibly skin biopsies, to confirm a diagnosis of scleroderma. But such tests aren't definitive. Scleroderma symptoms vary and may come and go, especially in milder cases, making the disease difficult to diagnose.

Because there is no cure for scleroderma, treatments are meant to relieve symptoms. For example, blood pressure drugs that relax the constriction of blood vessels can help ease Raynaud's syndrome, and acid-lowering drugs can ease heartburn symptoms. NSAIDs or other painkillers help treat muscle pain. Hand therapy for scleroderma includes stretching and range-of-motion exercises, gentle massage and splinting to reduce joint contractures, home paraffin treatments to soften skin, and help with modifying routine activities to limit stress on tender joints and relieve joint pain and swelling (see "Getting a grip: Handy gadgets and advice," page 47).

Psoriatic arthritis

This uncommon type of arthritis is related to psoriasis, a chronic skin condition marked by thick, red patches of skin covered with silvery scales. About a quarter of people with psoriasis develop psoriatic arthritis. In most cases, the skin condition is diagnosed first, but the arthritis may occur before the first signs of psoriasis, and some people with the condition have no skin lesions at all. Psoriatic arthritis can strike at any age but usually occurs between the ages of 20 and 50.

The condition often affects the fingernails, causing small indentations (pitting) or lifting of the nails. As with all types of arthritis, joint swelling, stiffness, and pain are common; unlike rheumatoid arthritis, psori-

Continued on page 17

Cold hands: Is it Raynaud's syndrome?

If your fingers turn ghostly white and numb when exposed to cold, you may have Raynaud's syndrome. A common condition (it affects up to one in 10 people, most of them women), Raynaud's is an exaggeration of the body's normal response to cold. It usually affects the hands and feet and, less often, the nose, lips, and ears. Many people are extremely sensitive to the cold, but unless your extremities actually change color—to either white from lack of blood or blue from poorly oxygenated blood—you don't have Raynaud's.

When exposed to cold, the body normally slows its loss of heat and tries to preserve its core temperature. Blood vessels near the surface constrict, redirecting blood flow deeper into the body. In Raynaud's, this process is more extreme and can occur even with a fairly small decrease in air temperature.

An episode of Raynaud's begins when the blood vessels supplying the fingers and toes spasm and contract, hampering the flow of oxygen-rich blood to the skin. The skin becomes pale and cool, sometimes blanching to a stark white color. The affected tissues may become numb and cold, and people with Raynaud's are more susceptible to frostbite than other people. However, a key feature of Raynaud's is that it is reversible. When the blood vessels relax and blood flow resumes, the skin becomes warm and flushed—and very red. The fingers or toes may throb or tingle.

Some people with Raynaud's have other health problems, usually connective tissue disorders such as scleroderma or lupus. Your doctor can determine this by doing a physical exam, asking you about your symptoms, and running a few blood tests. But most of the time, there is no underlying medical problem.

The best treatment for Raynaud's is to prevent episodes, mainly by avoiding sudden and unprotected exposure to cold temperatures. Keeping your whole body warm helps prevent the reflexive constriction of blood vessels in your skin. Before you head outside into the cold, put on gloves and warm footwear, but also bundle up your entire body and head, taking advantage of items such as long underwear, vests, lightweight activewear, and even single-use hand warmers. Preheat your car before getting in. You may want to wear gloves in chilly grocery store aisles and when reaching into your own freezer, if you find that action triggers the problem. Even exposure to air conditioning may be troublesome for people with Raynaud's.

It's also a good idea to avoid other things that cause your blood vessels to constrict. Smoking is one such aggravating factor. Certain medications may also constrict the blood vessels; these include amphetamines, cold and allergy formulas that contain phenylephrine or pseudoephedrine, and migraine drugs that contain ergotamine. Stressful events may also provoke an episode of Raynaud's. After a large meal, blood is diverted from the extremities to the digestive system, so keep food intake moderate.

Relaxation techniques can help prevent stress-induced episodes. Thermal biofeedback, which trains people to self-regulate their finger temperature, also shows some promise in treating Raynaud's. This technique uses sensors placed on the fingers that feed temperature information to a video screen, so you can monitor your progress.

Your doctor may prescribe a medication that relaxes the blood vessels, usually a calcium-channel blocker. If it's not effective, other blood pressure drugs that open up blood vessels may help. Drugs used to treat erectile dysfunction (which work by expanding blood vessels and boosting blood flow) have been found to have a moderate effect in easing Raynaud's symptoms. You may not need to take these drugs all the time, but only during the cold season, when Raynaud's tends to be worse.

In severe cases that have not responded to other therapy, case reports indicate that injections of botulinum toxin A (Botox, Dysport, Xeomin) may improve blood flow in the fingers and reduce symptoms. Research trials are ongoing.

If drug treatment fails to provide adequate relief of symptoms, a surgical procedure called sympathectomy is an option. Surgical sympathectomy removes the small nerves that surround the blood vessels of the hands and fingers. These nerves belong to the sympathetic nervous system, which orchestrates the fight-or-flight response, and they make the neighboring blood vessels constrict. Removing the nerves allows maximum dilation of these vessels.

Once a Raynaud's episode starts, it's important to get warm as quickly as possible. Try soaking your hands in lukewarm (about 105° F) water, or put them under your armpits or in another warm area. But don't put your hands, feet, or face on a heater or anything else that could scald or otherwise injure you.

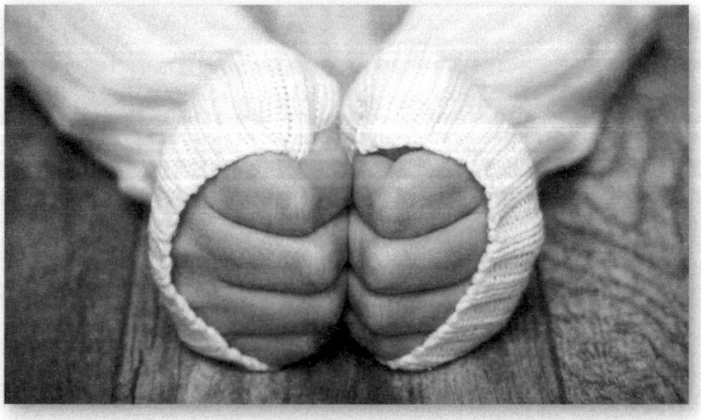

If your hands don't change color—to either white from lack of blood or blue from poorly oxygenated blood—you don't have Raynaud's. The hands shown here are just normal cold hands.

Continued from page 15
atic arthritis usually affects only a few joints and tends to be asymmetric (that is, joints on both sides of the body are not necessarily affected similarly). Diagnosis is based on the person's history of psoriasis; physical examination of the skin, nails, and joints; x-rays; and, in some cases, tests of fluid from the joints.

Treatments for psoriatic arthritis include those used for rheumatoid arthritis, such as oral and injected steroids, topical and oral NSAIDs, and DMARDs (see Table 1, page 8; Table 2, page 9; and Table 3, page 13). One DMARD (apremilast) is approved specifically for psoriatic arthritis.

In a 2020 publication, researchers compared hand function in rheumatoid arthritis and psoriatic arthritis and found similar reductions in grip strength, fine motor control, and people's perceptions of their hand function over time. Hand therapy treatments that can help include reducing activity, protecting the joint, controlling swelling, improving range of motion, and learning gentle stretching and strengthening techniques.

Symptoms of psoriatic arthritis

- ✔ Joint swelling, stiffness, and pain in one or more joints
- ✔ Pitting of the fingernails and toenails
- ✔ In some cases, silver or gray scaly spots on the scalp, elbows, knees, or lower spine

Joint reconstruction for arthritic hands

Replacing knee, hip, and shoulder joints is almost routine these days. Replacing hand joints is less common but quite similar, just on a smaller scale. Advances in materials and mechanics have made replacing hand joints—including the entire wrist, as well as knuckle and finger joints—a viable option. The need for artificial hand joints has declined somewhat in recent years, thanks to the success of drug treatments (especially DMARDs) in keeping crippling inflammatory arthritis of the hands at bay. But joint replacement remains an important option for many people.

Thumb surgery

The hand joint most commonly operated on is the basal joint, also called the first carpometacarpal (CMC) joint, located at the base of the thumb where it meets the wrist (see Figure 1, page 3). The surgery, called CMC arthroplasty, is usually done in people with osteoarthritis to treat pain, loss of function, or both. Appearance may be a secondary factor.

One of several techniques can be used. The surgeon removes all or part of the trapezium (the irregularly shaped bone at the base of the thumb) and then stabilizes your thumb, often using one of your own tendons to provide support. Sometimes a tendon is used as a sling to support the thumb, and other times the tendon is used

Figure 4: Surgery for arthritis in the thumb

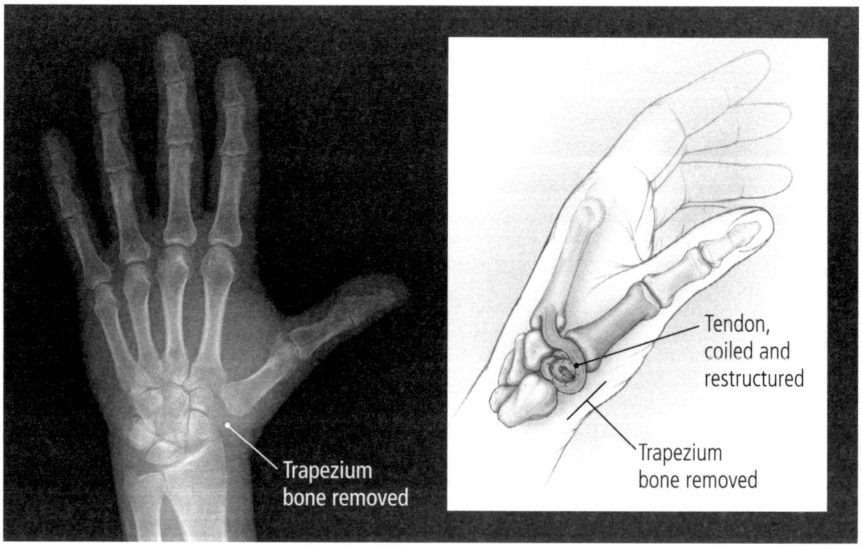

Total joint reconstruction is a common type of surgery for arthritis in the basal or first carpometacarpal (CMC) joint. The surgeon removes the arthritic trapezium bone (see the x-ray on the left) and then uses a nearby tendon to stabilize the thumb base. Sometimes the tendon is arranged as a sling, and other times it's used as a cushion in the space that remains when the trapezium is removed (see the illustration on the right). Because soft tissues are not visible on an x-ray, the tendon does not show up on the x-ray image.

Recovery may take several months, but the goal is the return of functional, pain-free joint motion and pinching and gripping strength as well as pain relief. Generally, this is a highly successful operation with few complications and excellent long-term results.

to create a cushion that fits into the space where the trapezium once resided (see Figure 4, page 18). The surgeon can also use a fiber cable to help stabilize the thumb (see "Stephen's story," at right). Implanting an artificial prosthetic joint is less common, and studies have shown higher rates of failure.

Wrist surgery: Total joint replacement vs. fusion

Total joint replacement (arthroplasty) involves removing damaged bone or joints and replacing them with a prosthetic joint. It is intended primarily to reduce pain while allowing for some range of motion, which may make everyday tasks like writing and hair combing much easier. Prosthetic joints may be made from silicone, polyethylene, titanium, or pyrocarbon, a substance consisting of a tough, ceramic-like coating over graphite.

People with rheumatoid arthritis are the most likely candidates for a total wrist replacement. About two-thirds of people with rheumatoid arthritis have wrist symptoms within two years of their diagnosis, and that number rises to more than 90% by 10 years (see "Should you consider a joint replacement?" on page 20). People with osteoarthritis or post-traumatic arthritis (a form of arthritis resulting from a previous fracture or ligament injury) may also benefit from the procedure.

Wrist replacement can be done under either general or regional block anesthesia as an inpatient or outpatient procedure. The surgeon removes the first row of carpal (wrist) bones and shapes the end of the radius (the main forearm bone) to fit the prosthesis. The radial component of the prosthesis inserts into the radius, while the carpal component inserts into the remaining carpal bones. A plastic spacer fits between the two components (see Figure 5, page 20).

Wrist fusion surgery is another option for treating a painful, arthritic wrist. The surgeon removes any remaining cartilage from the bone of the wrist and then typically stabilizes the wrist with a long metal plate which holds the bones in position while they fuse together to form a single bone.

There are different risks and benefits to wrist replacement and wrist fusion surgery. Replacement allows for some motion at the wrist but typically is not as durable as fusion and may require additional surgery in the future, while fusion provides reliable stability and healing but does not allow for wrist motion.

A failed wrist replacement—in which an implant loosens and pain and deformity occur—can be redone as a wrist fusion, but it is a challenging operation that requires bone grafting to fill the space formerly occupied by the implant.

After wrist replacement surgery, you'll first wear a plaster forearm splint, which is applied in the operating room, for about

STEPHEN'S STORY: Thumb surgery

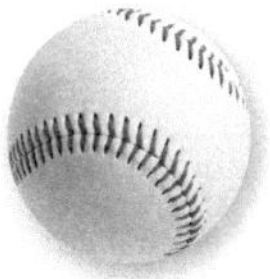

A lifelong athlete, Stephen, now 72, wanted to keep playing softball during his summers in New Hampshire and winters in Florida. But he had developed thumb arthritis that made it difficult to keep enjoying his sport. This is his story:

Arthritis in my thumb bothered me for over 20 years. I had gutted and renovated 13 houses and played softball and lots of basketball over the years, so that was probably hard on my hands. Besides hoping to continue playing softball, what drove me to get it fixed was when I couldn't ride a bike without pain and couldn't swing a hammer at all because it hurt so much.

I consulted a surgeon who was very nice, but after cortisone shots didn't help, he wanted to fuse my wrist and thumb. He said, "If you were my father, I would fuse this and tell you to go fishing." That meant I wasn't going to be doing anything I loved, so I started looking for someone else to help me.

In Boston, the surgeon was doing a fairly new procedure that involved removing the trapezium bone to take the pain away and inserting a fiber cable from my thumb to a bone in my index finger. My surgery was in November, and she made me promise not to play softball until February. During that time, I wore a customized brace from a hand therapist and was able to start lifting and working out while wearing it.

This has been life-changing for me. My wrist looks a little weird because there is some bone missing, but my grip strength is back, and I can throw a ball as hard as I used to.

Should you consider a joint replacement?

Joint replacement is always an elective procedure. Although your surgeon may make you aware of the possibility of joint replacement, you must weigh the benefits and risks and come to your own decision about whether, or when, to undergo this major surgery.

Although age is an important factor, the decision to have a joint replacement is based on your disability—that is, how much pain you are in and how much your joint problems limit your activities. Joint surgery, either fusion or replacement, may be a good option if one or more of the following apply to you:

- You are unable to complete normal daily tasks without help.
- You have significant pain every day.
- Pain keeps you awake at night despite the use of medications.
- Nonsurgical approaches such as medications and splints have not relieved your pain.
- Less-complicated surgical procedures are unlikely to help.
- Pain keeps you from doing daily activities or your job.
- Pain doesn't subside when you rest.
- You are suffering severe side effects from the medications needed to control your joint symptoms.

Figure 5: Wrist replacement (arthroplasty)

In a wrist replacement, a surgeon replaces the damaged wrist joint with an artificial joint that includes several metal components. The radial component inserts into the radius bone, while the carpal component is secured into the carpal bones with one long stem and two screws. A polyethylene (plastic) spacer fits between the other two components in the joint area. Flat on one side and rounded on the other, the spacer's design allows it to fit into the carpal component while it rocks on the radial component, enabling a natural wrist motion.

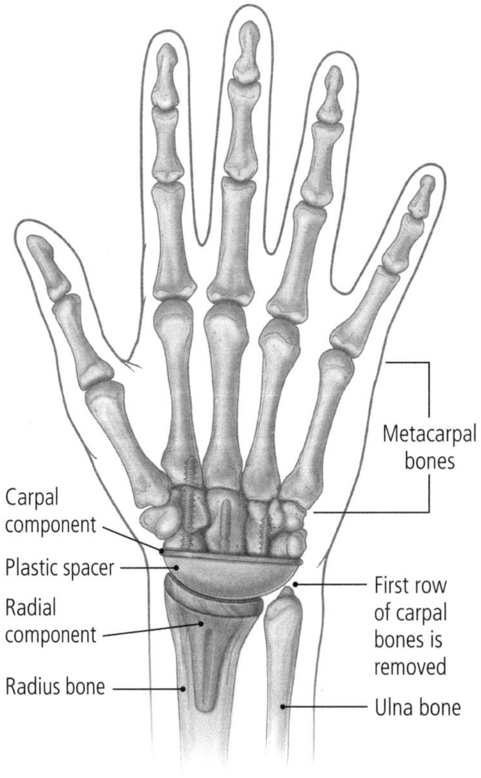

10 days. Then a hand therapist will make a customized splint that you'll use for four to six weeks. For wrist fusion surgery, you will need to wear a splint for 10 days followed by a cast for four weeks. During your recovery, you should work with a certified hand therapist, who can help you control the pain and swelling from the surgery. She or he will recommend specific exercises (see "Exercises for the hands," page 43) and teach you how to safely grip and support items to avoid putting undue stress on your wrist. (Also see "Surgical scars," page 21, for tips on making your scars less noticeable.)

Surgery on finger joints

In rheumatoid arthritis of the hand, the joints most commonly affected are the knuckles (the MCP joints). When this happens, it often leads to the disfiguring displacement of the fingers known as ulnar deviation, in which the fingers angle away from the thumb. Joint replacement is possible, but challenging, since the MCP joints in all the fingers but the thumb are shallow ball-and-socket joints that rely on tendons and ligaments to keep them stable. This means that reconstruction of both the tendons and ligaments is an essential part of the procedure (see Figure 6, page 21). Still, surgeons have used silicone and silastic (a blend of silicone and plastic) spacers to replace damaged MCP joints. While long-term follow-up shows some deterioration of the reconstructed joints, very few people require additional surgery to correct this. Pyrocarbon MCP joint implants can also be used, but these require intact, stable ligaments, which precludes their use in many patients.

As with MCP joints, surgeons have used both silicone and pyrocarbon implants to replace the PIP, or middle, joint of the finger. A pyrocarbon PIP joint replacement was approved by the FDA in 2002 as a Humanitarian Use Device (for conditions or diseases that typically affect fewer than 4,000 people in the United States per year). However, pyrocarbon joint implants are controversial, with nearly a quarter of recipients undergoing additional surgery to correct problems within six years. For this reason, your surgeon may recommend a silicone replacement or a fusion procedure (see Figure 7, page 22).

Fusion of the PIP joint is an accepted and frequently suggested procedure with a low complication rate. Although the joint can't be bent following surgery, for many people that is an acceptable tradeoff for the complete relief of pain.

For the DIP joint, fusion is realistically the only procedure. It has a low complication rate and high success rate.

Preparing for hand surgery

Recovering from any surgery is hard, but making do with just one hand for several weeks (or longer) poses some additional challenges. Taking time to prepare in advance can ease some of the inconvenience. Also, remember to pace yourself after surgery and avoid straining or injuring your other hand or arm.

Get organized. Contact your insurance company in advance about coverage for the surgical procedure, follow-up office visits, and therapy visits. Make a folder to organize your bills, appointment reminders, and postoperative recommendations. Ask your doctor for an estimated recovery time,

Figure 6: Surgery to correct hand deformities

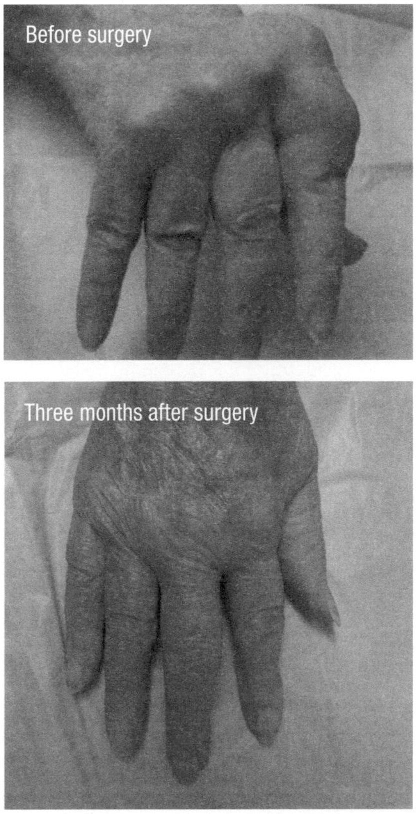

Much of the deformity caused by rheumatoid arthritis can be surgically corrected. This woman had arthroplasty of the MCP joints in her right hand plus reconstructive surgery. The surgeon removed diseased joint tissue, replaced it with silicone implants, rearranged soft tissue, and reconstructed ligaments.

Photos reprinted with permission, Barry P. Simmons, M.D.

Surgical scars

All surgeries have the potential to leave scars, but you can take steps to make them less noticeable. Most surgical dressings are removed within seven to 10 days. Your scar may be red and bumpy, but it will eventually lighten and flatten. Provided the wound is completely closed and has no drainage, you can try these tips to minimize the appearance of a scar:

- Gently massage the scar with a nonallergenic cream or lotion (such as Eucerin cream) two to three times per day. The motions should be circular, side to side, and up and down.
- If your scar is raised (known as a hypertrophic scar), use a scar pad (available in drugstores), which places gentle pressure on the scar to help flatten it.
- Use sunscreen (at least SPF 15) to prevent the scar from becoming darker.
- Gentle stretching can also help, but it depends on the location of the scar.

See a certified hand therapist for recommendations for specific exercises and other advice about your particular scars. It typically takes up to a year after an injury or surgery for a scar to stop changing in appearance.

Figure 7: Finger joint repair: Replacement vs. fusion

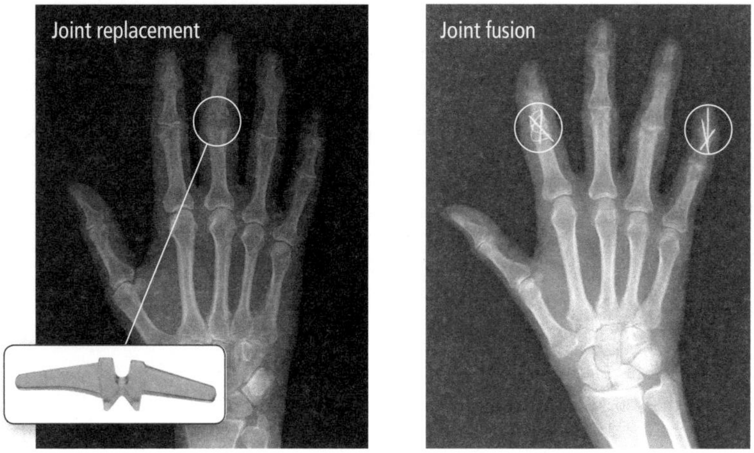

The x-ray on the left shows an example of PIP joint replacement in the middle finger. It uses a silicone joint (inset) that allows the finger to bend. Because the implant is not metal (unlike the image on the right), it does not show up prominently on the x-ray.

The x-ray on the right shows joint fusion in the PIP joint of the index finger and the DIP joint of the small finger. The surgery required bone grafts, pins, and wires to hold the joints in place.

Whether fusion or replacement is better for you depends on your individual case. Joint fusions have a high success rate and provide a pain-free, stable, but unmovable joint. Joint replacements allow movement and provide good pain relief, but are less reliable, meaning a repeat procedure may be needed.

X-rays reprinted with permission, Brandon E. Earp, M.D., and Barry P. Simmons, M.D. Inset photo courtesy Smith & Nephew.

so you can talk to your employer about when you'll be able to return to work. Set up automatic bill payments, or pay bills ahead of time.

Ask for help. Enlist help in advance from family, friends, or neighbors. Get a small calendar to keep track of who will be available when. Update their phone and email addresses and keep them handy. You may need assistance with transportation to and from surgery and follow-up appointments; caring for children, pets, and plants; and doing yard work and housecleaning. Consider hiring a cleaning service, even for just one or two visits.

Modify your self-care. Practice dressing and undressing, using the bathroom, showering, and brushing and flossing your teeth with one hand. Useful tools include shampoo and toothpaste in flip-top or pump dispensers, prestrung dental flossers, and an electric toothbrush. Keep a hairbrush in the shower to assist with shampooing. Buy a terry cloth robe for drying yourself after bathing or showering. You may need to keep your hand dry and wrap it after surgery, so check your drugstore or look online for cast protectors.

Eat efficiently. Prepare meals ahead and freeze them. Buy frozen, microwaveable dinners. Plan for "no cut" meals such as sandwiches, ground meat, and finger foods. Make a contact list of favorite takeout and delivery options. Stock up on nonperishables. Use fewer dishes (or paper plates), so you don't have so many to wash.

Simplify your wardrobe. Loose clothing and elastic-waist pants will ease the task of getting dressed. Avoid clothes with buttons and zippers. Slip-on shoes are a good idea, too.

Tendon trouble

Think of the tendons in your arms and hands as the strings of a marionette, enabling you to lift your wrist and hand and to move your thumb and fingers. For a variety of reasons or for no apparent reason, the tendons or tendon sheaths can become inflamed, causing pain whenever you put any tension on the tendon. Certain tendons and tendon sheaths in the fingers, wrists, and elbows are particularly prone to inflammation, leading to specific types of tendinitis, tenosynovitis, and epicondylitis.

De Quervain's tendinitis

Tendinitis is swelling of the tendon. In the wrist, the most common location for tendinitis is on the thumb side. When it occurs there, it is called de Quervain's tendinitis (also known as tenosynovitis). De Quervain's results from repetitive hand and wrist movements—for example, while gardening or playing sports. It is sometimes called "new mother's disease" because it often develops in women with newborn babies, possibly as a result of repetitive movements made while caring for an infant. But new fathers, grandparents, and other caregivers can also experience these symptoms.

The main symptom is pain over the thumb side of the wrist, which can appear gradually or suddenly and may move up the forearm. The pain worsens when you grasp things or twist your wrist. Picking up a coffee mug may cause exquisite pain. You may notice swelling over the affected tendon, and a fluid-filled cyst may arise in the same area. The thumb may occasionally "catch" or "snap" when you move it.

To diagnose de Quervain's, the doctor checks for tenderness over the tendons on the thumb side of the wrist. He or she may ask you to make a fist with your fingers over the thumb and bend your wrist toward the little finger. This maneuver, known as the Finkelstein test, is usually quite painful for a person with de Quervain's.

Treatments include resting the thumb and wrist by wearing a splint (see "Splints," page 24). Your doctor may also recommend anti-inflammatory medicines to curb pain and reduce swelling. Steroid injections into the tendon compartment may help. In a 2016 analysis of results from six previous studies, the combination of splinting plus steroid injections was more successful at treating de Quervain's than either approach on its own. If all these measures fail to improve your symptoms, surgery (which releases the tight tendon sheath) is often successful. A hand therapist can design an exercise program to restore flexibility and strength once the initial symptoms clear up.

Trigger finger

The medical condition called trigger finger has nothing to do with weapons, nor does it occur primarily in the index finger, as the name would imply. Instead, this ailment—officially known as stenosing tenosynovitis—is most common in the ring finger and the

Continued on page 25

Symptoms of de Quervain's tendinitis

- ✔ Pain on the thumb side of the wrist, especially when pinching, grasping, or making a fist
- ✔ A small knot or tenderness on the thumb side of the wrist

Symptoms of trigger finger (or thumb)

- ✔ Pain and sometimes swelling where the finger or thumb meets the palm
- ✔ When you bend or straighten the affected digit, it may catch and then suddenly release

Splints

The basic purpose of a splint is to immobilize an injured or inflamed part of the body, allowing it to heal. Splints can provide pain relief, allow you to function, or realign your joints better. Certified hand therapists are trained to assess your hand and choose or fabricate a splint to meet your needs.

Splints come in a wide range of materials and forms. Prefabricated splints from the drugstore or a medical supply store (such as splints 2 and 3—the MetaGrip and Comfort Cool, respectively) work well to restore function for people with arthritis of the CMC joint of the thumb, provided you choose and adjust the splint correctly. Other conditions require specially fabricated splints, which are usually made of thermoplastic materials and molded to fit around the contours of your hand (splints 1, 4, and 5). Silver ring splints, which look like jewelry, are flexible and strong and can be worn on the fingers during most activities to treat trigger finger and various other problems in thumb and finger joints (splint 6). These splints are ordered after you are measured by a hand therapist. Less expensive finger splints are available in other materials and are fitted and issued to the patient by the hand therapist. For people with rheumatoid arthritis, resting hand splints keep joints in a neutral position to minimize your pain and prevent muscle shortening and joint deformity (splint 7).

Static splints (all seven shown here) hold a joint in one position. Dynamic splints (not pictured) allow for movement. Some are designed to help lengthen tightened joint capsules, muscles, and tendons. Others, which feature elastic or spring-loaded parts, allow a significantly weakened hand or wrist to move after a tendon or nerve injury.

Of course, a splint only works if you have the right type for your specific problem and if you use it correctly. For example, splints used to treat carpal tunnel syndrome (splint 4) are intended to be worn only when you're sleeping or resting—not when you're using your wrist. Some common complaints about splints are that they don't look good, they immobilize too many joints (which limits your ability to function), or they fit poorly (which can cause pressure and irritate the skin). If you're having any of these problems, consult a therapist.

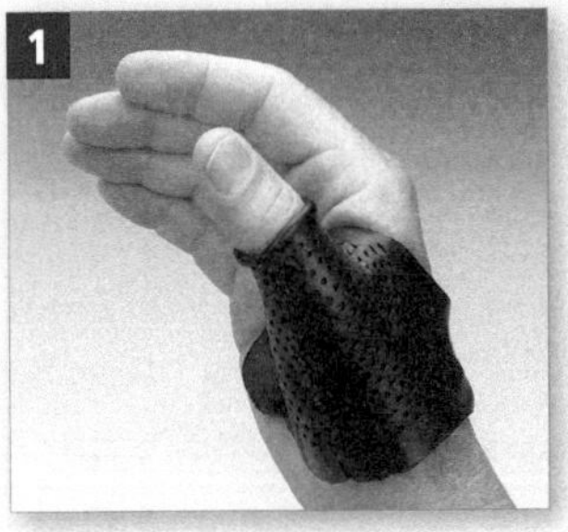

A custom-made short opponens splint immobilizes the thumb only and can help ease the pain of thumb osteoarthritis while allowing hand function.

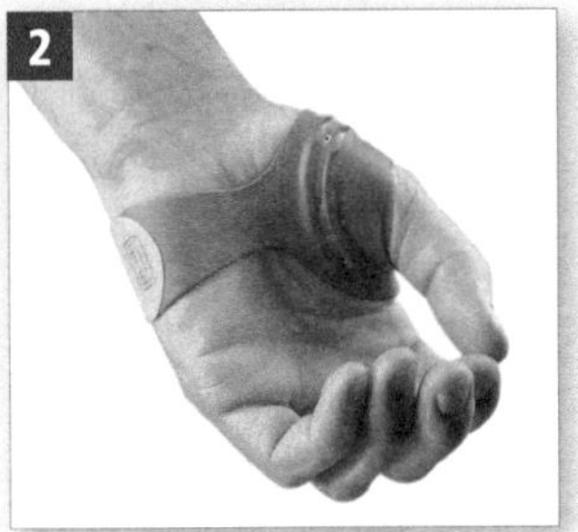

A semi-rigid brace supports the base of the thumb to ease osteoarthritis pain, but allows for light to moderate function.

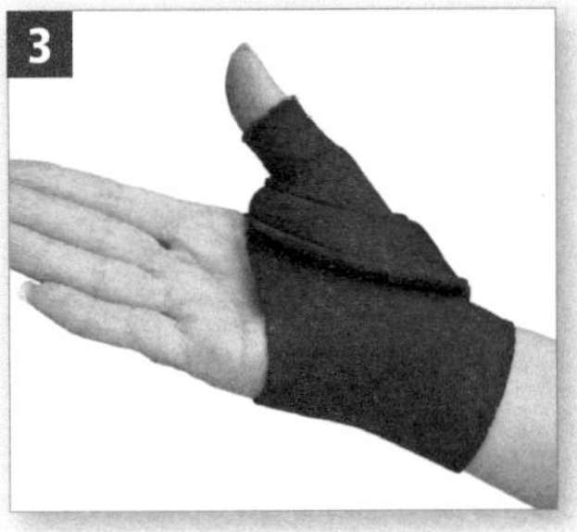

A soft functional splint provides gentle support to the thumb and still allows you to use your hand for light activities.

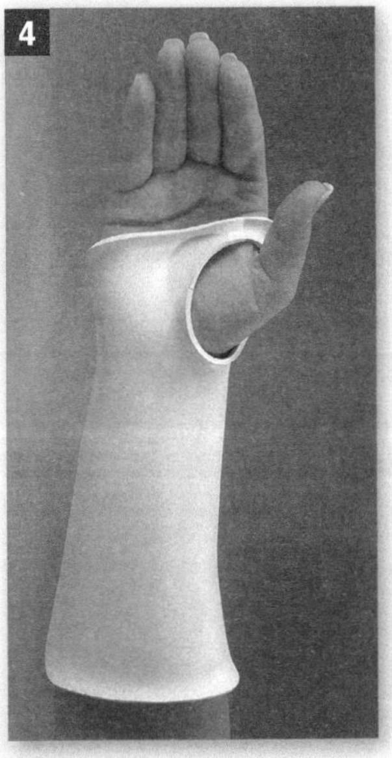

A wrist immobilizer holds the wrist straight, in a neutral position, which helps people with carpal tunnel syndrome. It is used when the hand is at rest. To treat tennis elbow, this type of splint may also be configured with the wrist tilted up to reduce tension on the extensor tendons.

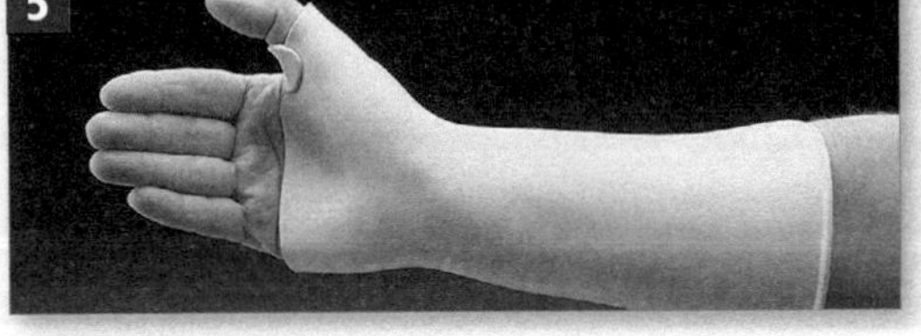

A custom-made long opponens splint, often recommended for de Quervain's tendinitis, immobilizes both the thumb and wrist.

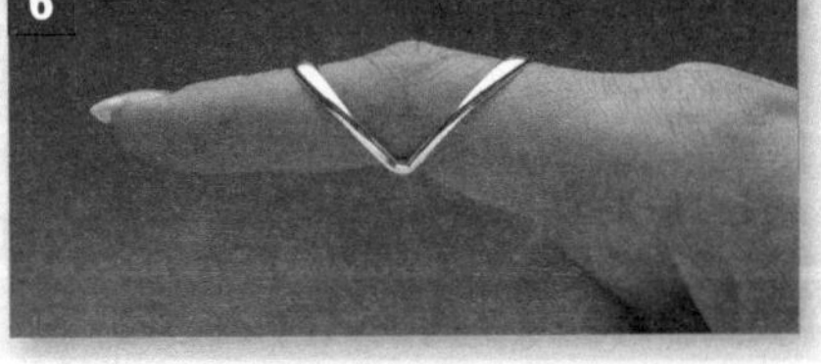

A silver ring splint blocks hyperextension of the middle joint of the finger to correct a swan-neck deformity.

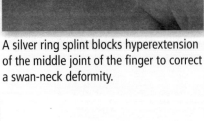

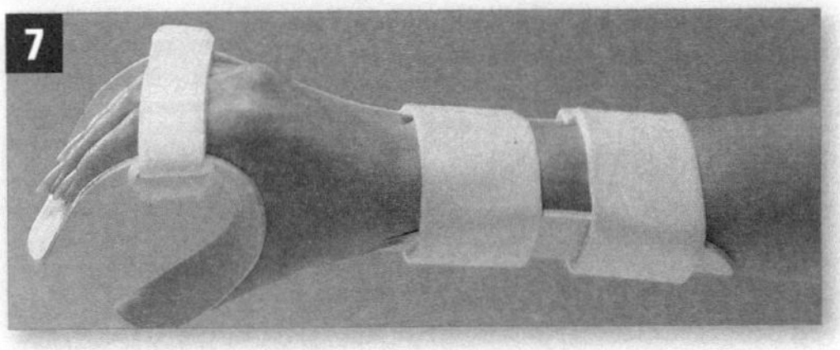

A resting hand splint, sometimes recommended for rheumatoid arthritis, minimizes ulnar deviation.

Photos 1,4,5, and 7: Performance Health. Photo 2: BraceLab. Photo 3: North Coast Medical. Photo 6: Silver Ring Splints.

Continued from page 23
thumb. It is called trigger finger because of the trigger-like snap that occurs when the finger briefly locks and then suddenly releases when you try to bend or straighten it. The condition affects the tendons that bend the fingers and the pulleys (rings of connective tissue) that hold those tendons close to the finger bones (see Figure 8, below). If the tendon develops a knot (nodule) or if the lining covering the tendon swells, it has to squeeze through the opening of the tunnel, causing pain, popping, or a catching feeling in the finger or thumb. When the tendon catches, the pulley also becomes swollen and irritated, creating a vicious cycle. Sometimes the tendon becomes stuck in the pulley and the finger can't be straightened or bent. It's like having a knot in your shoelace: if the knot is small, it catches only briefly when it passes through the eyelet of the shoe; if the knot is large, it can get stuck and cannot pass through the eyelet.

Trigger finger or thumb often starts with a sense of discomfort at the base of the digit, which may also thicken slightly. If the finger begins to trigger or lock, you may think the problem is at the middle knuckle of the finger or the top knuckle of the thumb, but it's actually inflammation of the pulley at the base of the affected finger. It's not clear what causes trigger finger, but people who are older than 40 and who have rheumatoid arthritis, gout, or diabetes seem to be more susceptible to the problem.

Wearing a splint, taking anti-inflammatory drugs, and getting a steroid injection in the area around the tendon can all help break the cycle of inflammation and pain. If your symptoms don't improve, surgery is an option.

The operation—a quick procedure that takes only about 10 minutes—opens the pulley, allowing the tendon to glide through it more easily. Usually, this restores finger movement right away, although some people feel tenderness, swelling, and discomfort for four to six weeks, or possibly longer. A full recovery, meaning your finger feels back to normal, often takes at least three months and can take up to a full year.

Figure 8: Trigger finger

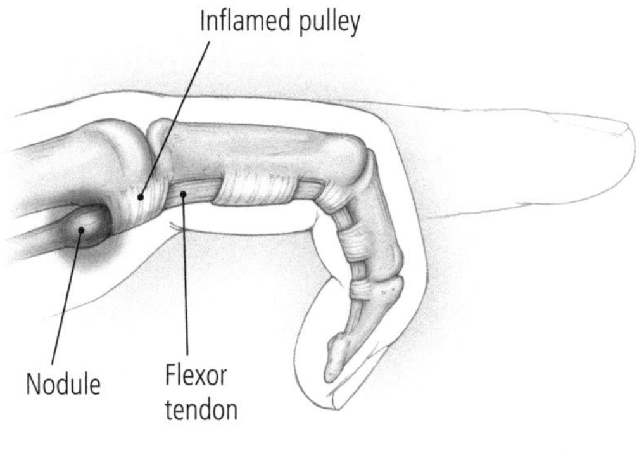

An often-painful condition, trigger finger is caused by a narrowing of the sheath that surrounds the tendon and irritation of the pulley, the ring of connective tissue that holds the tendon close to the bone. Trigger finger is most common in people over age 40. Symptoms include a sensation of "catching" when trying to bend or straighten the finger. A bump (nodule) may also form.

Tennis elbow

Why include tennis elbow in a report on hands? Also known as lateral epicondylitis or lateral elbow tendinopathy, this condition involves degenerative changes of the fibers that attach your forearm muscles to the outside of the elbow. These muscles lift the wrist and hand. So, every time you use your hand, the tendon attached to your elbow hurts. You may feel mild pain in your outer elbow that gradually worsens over weeks and months, becoming a severe, burning pain. Pressing the outside of the elbow or lifting even very light objects, like a book or coffee cup, can hurt.

Although the problem can occur in people of all ages, it's most common between the ages of 30 and 50. Despite the name, most people with tennis elbow don't play tennis or other racquet sports. They might be involved in work or other activities that require them to use their forearm muscles in repetitive, vigorous ways—shoveling snow, for example. But most have no apparent reason for developing symptoms.

Symptoms of tennis elbow

- ✔ Pain on the outer side of the elbow and down the forearm, usually in your dominant arm
- ✔ Worsening of pain if you straighten your wrist or try to pick up a heavy object

Treatment focuses first on easing pain. Reducing activity and putting ice on your elbow can help, as can anti-inflammatory medications. Your doctor or hand therapist may also recommend certain braces or splints that allow your tendons and muscles to rest and heal (see "Splints," page 24). Kinesiotape (below) is an increasingly popular option. Massage and other soft-tissue techniques and pain-free stretching and strengthening exercises may be added to your regimen as your treatment progresses. The exercise program may also include strengthening of your shoulder and core to improve your overall mobility and function.

Your symptoms should improve within six to eight weeks, although complete healing may take as long as 12 to 15 months. A therapist can teach you specific exercises to strengthen the affected muscles and show you how to modify your activities so your symptoms don't return. Most people are able to recover over time with these conservative treatments. But one in 10 patients ends up needing surgery to remove damaged tendon tissue and reattach normal tendon tissue to bone.

Golfer's elbow

You can also develop degenerative changes on the inside of your elbow; this is known medically as medial epicondylitis. This condition usually arises from movements that involve turning the arm down and flexing the wrist, such as during a golf swing, which is why it's also known as golfer's elbow. But any activity that requires you to repeatedly bend your wrist or grip, grab, and turn your hand can cause the condition. The symptoms include tenderness and pain in the inner elbow, which worsen if you bend your wrist. The treatments resemble those for tennis elbow, but focus on the inner elbow.

Kinesiotape

You may have noticed athletes sporting colorful tape in various designs on their skin. Kinesiotape is thin, stretchy cotton tape with latex-free adhesive. Your therapist can show you how to use the tape, applied in a specific pattern, as an adjunct to your exercise program and hands-on therapy. It can reduce pain and swelling via stimulation through the skin, decrease spasms by helping muscles to relax, support muscles and joints without reducing your range of motion, lessen pressure on injured areas in between treatments, and help you sense when you are keeping your arms and hands in proper alignment. On the wrist and hands, therapists often use kinesiotape in therapy for such problems as tennis elbow, de Quervain's tendinitis, and finger sprains. A certified hand therapist can assess if kinesiotape would be beneficial to you and teach you how to properly apply it to get the desired benefits.

Symptoms of golfer's elbow

- ✔ Pain and tenderness in the inner elbow
- ✔ Worsening of pain if you bend your wrist

Dupuytren's disease

This uncommon hand problem is also known as Dupuytren's contracture because it causes the fingers to slowly contract and curl toward the palm. It results from an abnormal thickening of the fascia—the tissue between the skin and tendons—in the palm. Most people first notice a small lump in the palm, perhaps with some pitting or puckering of the skin. Some people later develop a tough cord beneath the skin stretching from the palm to the fingers, which prevents the fingers from fully straightening (see Figure 9, page 27).

Although no one knows exactly what causes Dupuytren's disease or why some people have worse contractures than others, it runs in families, suggesting that it has a genetic component. Named after the French surgeon who first treated the disease in 1830, Dupuytren's mostly affects people with Northern European heritage and is more common in men than women. Cigarette smoking, epilepsy, and diabetes may increase the risk for Dupuytren's.

The condition often begins near the base of the ring and little fingers. Dupuytren's disease usually doesn't hurt, but the initial nodules in the palm may be painful. Still, you might not notice the problem until months or even years later, when you find you cannot flatten the palm of your hand on a table or other flat surface. In a poem published in *JAMA*, a physician affected by the disease described his father's (and his own) experience with the deformity. He was "puzzled by the stinging and the curl of his fingers about a phantom hardball caught barehanded." In severe cases, when the fingers contract into the palm, it's difficult to do everyday activities such as washing your hands, putting on gloves, and sliding your hands into your pockets. With Dupuytren's, it's impossible to straighten the fingers, unlike a trigger finger, which can be intermittently straightened. Commonly, Dupuytren's affects both hands.

In the past, people with Dupuytren's disease were almost exclusively treated with surgery to release their bent fingers. Afterward, patients wore splints to keep their fingers straight, followed by therapy to ease swelling and help them regain finger function. But the thickened fascia and cord characteristic of this disease sometimes returned in the same place or elsewhere in the hand. A less invasive procedure called needle aponeurotomy or percutaneous fasciotomy, in which the doctor uses a small needle to divide and sever the contracting bands in the palm, yields similar results. This procedure is done under local anesthesia. People usually recover quickly, returning to normal activities within just a few days, without needing bandages or splints. However, despite the initial high success rate, the condition returns in up to 65% of patients.

In 2010, the FDA approved a nonsurgical treatment for Dupuytren's disease. Marketed under the name Xiaflex, the drug is made from an enzyme, called collagenase clostridium histolyticum, which breaks down the collagen fibers causing the contracture. Most of the time, the doctor treats only one finger at a time, with 30 days in between fingers. The doctor injects the medication directly into the collagen cord in your hand. Several days later, your hand is numbed and manipulated to release the cord (see Figure 10, page 28). Over the following one to three months, you wear a splint at night that holds your finger extended, and you perform exercises several times a day to maintain your finger's range of motion. The most common side effects include swelling, bleeding, and pain in the injected area. Sometimes the skin can tear where it has adhered to the Dupuytren's cord, but this is treated well with dressings. In rare cases, the collagenase can leak into the tendon, causing it to rupture—a serious complication.

Figure 9: Anatomy of Dupuytren's contracture

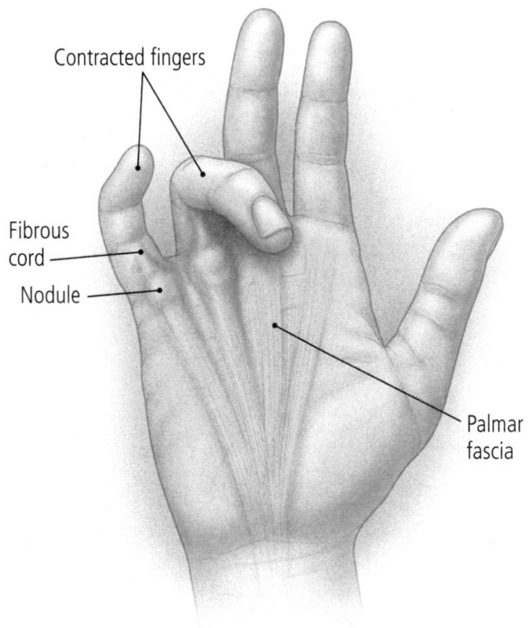

A contracture from Dupuytren's disease develops when the palmar fascia (the tissue overlying the tendons in the palm) shortens and contracts, pulling the fingers inward. The first sign may be a nodule near the crease of the hand below the finger. A fibrous cord may develop that extends from the palm to the finger.

In a study published in *The New England Journal of Medicine*, 308 people with contractures involving joints of the ring or little finger received injections of either Xiaflex or a placebo. The following day, the investigators manually extended the fingers (as much as the patients could tolerate) to break the cord and release the contracture. Subjects could receive up to three injections (at intervals of about one month). Nearly 85% of joints injected with collagenase showed some improvement, and 64% were straight or nearly

Symptoms of Dupuytren's disease

- ✔ Small lump or pit in the palm crease closest to the ring and little fingers
- ✔ Inability to flatten the palm on an even surface
- ✔ Fingers may eventually curl toward the palm

Figure 10: Before and after collagenase treatment of Dupuytren's contracture

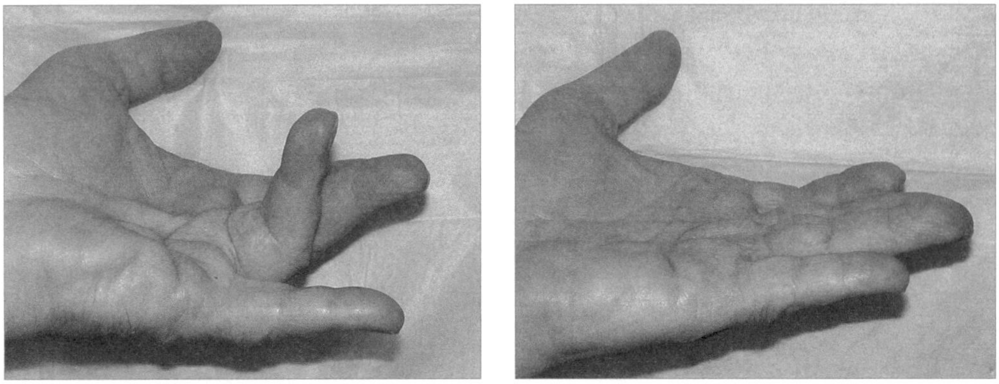

At left, severe contractures of the ring and middle fingers in a person with Dupuytren's disease before treatment with injectable collagenase (Xiaflex). At right, the same hand several months after treatment.

Photos reprinted with permission, Barry P. Simmons, M.D.

straight, compared with 12% improved and 7% straight or nearly straight of those receiving placebo injections. Other studies show that after two years, recurrence rates were 14% for MCP joints and 23% for PIP joints.

Although all the treatments for Dupuytren's contracture are beneficial, none cure the disease. Three years after Xiaflex, recurrence is about 27% at the MCP joint and 56% at the PIP joint. However, repeat injections are possible (see "Scott's story," page 29).

Ganglion cysts

If you notice a small, firm lump on the back of your wrist, at the base of a finger, or on the palm side of your wrist where you would take your pulse, don't be alarmed. Chances are it's a ganglion cyst—a common, harmless growth that develops from inside a joint, like a tiny balloon on a stalk (see Figure 11, at right). The balloon may be filled with fluid or a jelly-like substance and can usually be felt underneath the skin. The cyst may be painful and may wax and wane in size, sometimes growing as large as a peach pit. An old-time treatment for these cysts was to hit them with a heavy book, which is why they're also known as "Bible cysts." Don't try this, however—it's not effective, and you could fracture your wrist!

It's not clear what causes most ganglion cysts, although it is thought that flaws in the synovial lining of a joint allow the synovial fluid to form a fluid-filled cyst that can change shape. They're more common in women than in men, and gymnasts (who often put a great deal of pressure on their wrists) seem to be especially susceptible to them.

Often, these cysts simply disappear with time. But if the cyst is painful, affects your daily activities, or is unattractive, you may want to consult a doctor. To diagnose the condition, the doctor will probably press on the cyst to check for tenderness or hold a penlight up to the cyst to see if the light shines through.

Because activity can cause the cyst to hurt, you

Symptoms of ganglion cyst

- ✔ Small, firm lump on the wrist or hand that is usually painless, ranging in size from a pea to a peach pit
- ✔ Lumps may disappear and reappear

Figure 11: Ganglion cyst

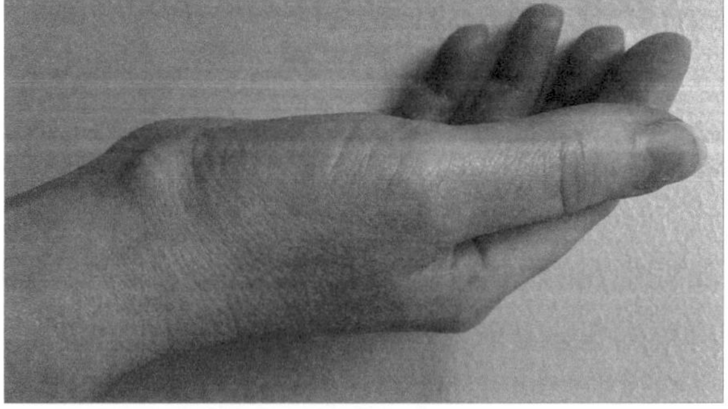

A volar ganglion cyst appears on the palm side of the wrist. Ganglion cysts on the back of the wrist are called dorsal cysts.

Photo reprinted with permission, Brandon E. Earp, M.D.

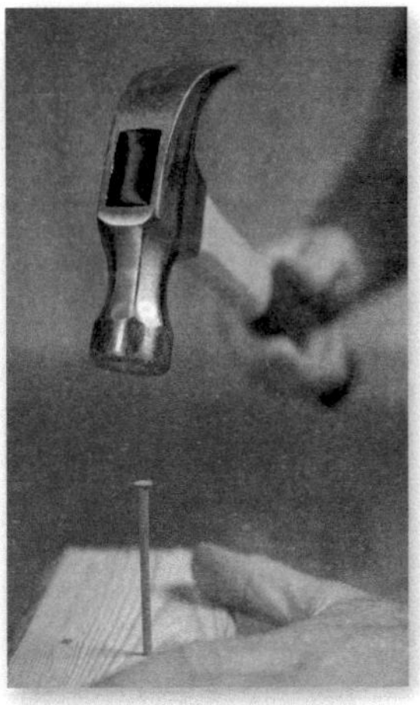

SCOTT'S STORY:
Injections and surgery for Dupuytren's disease

Having played football in high school and college, Scott, now 70, was no stranger to painful hand injuries, including a broken finger. But it was not pain that led him to consult a hand surgeon; it was the worsening curling of the fingers of both his hands. This is his story:

It progressed the same in both hands. First my little finger and then ring finger started to curl to the point where I couldn't put my hand in my pocket or hold a football. I couldn't put on gloves unless they were really stretchy and oversized. At my biotech job I had trouble typing on the keyboard because I couldn't extend my fingers properly. I met lots of new people because of my job, but my little and ring fingers were so curved that I couldn't shake hands. People thought I was doing something weird, and it was embarrassing. Just buttoning a shirt became a problem, and it was difficult to grab on to a hammer, shovel, or rake.

The Dupuytren's started in my right hand, and those fingers were treated first with injections of collagenase [Xiaflex]. A few days later, while I held my hand up like I was saying "stop," the doctor bent my fingers back. The popping sound when the collagen cords were released was so startling, we laughed. It didn't hurt because lidocaine had been injected, but the enzyme that breaks down collagen also makes your skin more fragile, so there were a number of rips in my skin and I needed a couple of stitches. My hand was unusable for a week, and then I started hand therapy.

Improvement from the injections lasted about two years. After the Dupuytren's recurred, I had surgery on three fingers. After the outpatient procedure, my hand was bandaged and I was able to start hand therapy while the stitches were still in place. Obviously I have scars from the surgical incisions, but the recovery was really much quicker after surgery than the injections.

When the left hand worsened enough to do treatment, we went right to surgery. That's been almost a year, and it's been a dramatic improvement. I now have full mobility in all my fingers on both hands, no problems typing, and I can grab tools or footballs or baseballs.

If I had a friend with a doctor offering both options for treatment, I'd say go for the surgery. I thought the easier solution would be the Xiaflex, but it ultimately just delayed the surgery.

may be advised to wear a wrist splint (see photo, page 32) to relieve symptoms. After any pain or discomfort subsides, wrist-strengthening exercises may help (see "Exercises for the hands," page 43). Your doctor can also aspirate the cyst, which involves numbing the area and puncturing the cyst with a needle to draw out the fluid. But the cysts nearly always recur after aspiration. If the entire cyst is surgically removed, recurrence rate is about 10%. The surgery involves removing part of the affected joint capsule or tendon sheath. Recovery time varies, but you should be able to return to your daily activities within two to six weeks.

Carpal tunnel syndrome and other "pinched" nerves

Three major nerves travel from the spinal cord all the way to the hand: the median, ulnar, and radial nerves. Each is housed within passageways or tunnels, which may become narrowed for a variety of reasons. When that happens, it puts pressure on the nerve, causing symptoms such as numbness, tingling, clumsiness, or weakness in the hand.

The best-known and most common of these trapped or pinched nerve problems is carpal tunnel syndrome, which affects the median nerve as it passes through the wrist to the thumb, index, and middle fingers and the thumb side of the ring finger (see Figure 12, at right). A similar but far less common problem, known as cubital tunnel syndrome, occurs with compression of the ulnar nerve, which passes through the inner part of the elbow. Other nerves can also become entrapped, but such instances are very rare.

Carpal tunnel syndrome

The carpal tunnel consists of a U-shaped cluster of eight bones at the base of the palm. A strong ligament, called the transverse carpal ligament, arches across the bones, forming the roof of the tunnel. Within this tunnel lies the median nerve, which controls sensations in the palm side of the thumb, the index and middle fingers, and half of the ring finger. It also transmits the impulses to certain hand muscles that enable the fingers and thumb to move. If the carpal tunnel narrows, the resulting pressure decreases the blood supply to the nerve, causing carpal tunnel syndrome.

The classic symptoms are tingling or "pins and needles," numbness, pain, and clumsiness in the thumb and affected fingers. Often, these symptoms occur at night and awaken you from sleep. Sleeping with the wrists flexed—a common habit—can contribute to the nighttime symptoms. After you awaken, you may need to shake your hand to restore normal feeling. Some people say their hands feel swollen and useless, even though their hands don't appear swollen. As the condition progresses, you may start to feel tingling during the day, and the pain may radiate up your arm. It may become difficult to make a tight fist, grasp and manipulate small objects, or do other things with your hands. In severe, chronic cases, persistent numbness may occur, and the muscles at the base of

Figure 12: Carpal tunnel syndrome

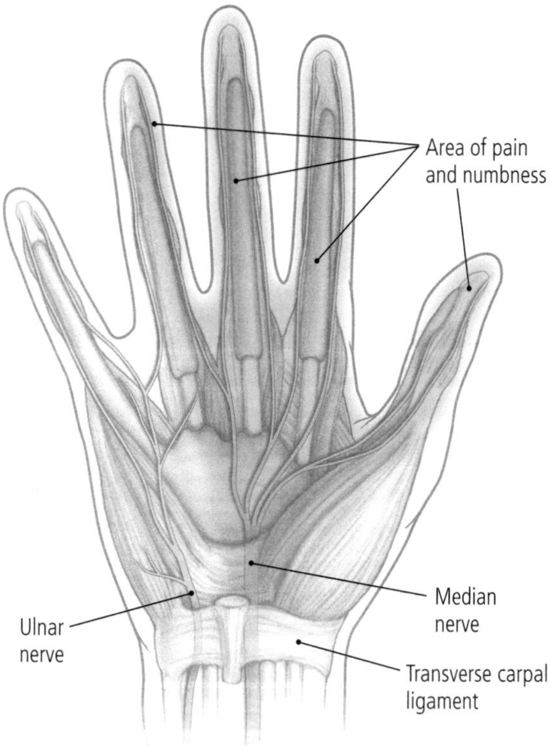

In carpal tunnel syndrome, the median nerve becomes compressed as it passes through the carpal tunnel, which is located on the palm side of the wrist. This narrow passage is formed by the transverse carpal ligament arching over a U-shaped cluster of eight bones. Pressure there causes numbness and tingling in the fingers served by the nerve. If you have carpal tunnel syndrome, it's important to seek evaluation early, as ongoing, increasing compression can lead to permanent nerve damage.

the thumb may weaken. You may even lose the ability to distinguish between hot and cold by touch.

Carpal tunnel syndrome affects about 3% of working adults. Women are three times as likely as men to have carpal tunnel syndrome, and the condition is most common in women over 50. It is not clear why some people get carpal tunnel syndrome and others don't. However, the following factors may contribute to the condition:

Heredity. Experts estimate that genes account for about half of cases. That assessment is based in part on studies that show a much higher risk in women who have an identical twin with the disorder compared with those with a fraternal twin. (Identical twins have all of the same genes, while fraternal twins have fewer genes in common.)

Tunnel size. Although the size of your wrist doesn't seem to matter, having a smaller carpal tunnel may make you more prone to the problem. This may help explain why women are more likely than men to develop carpal tunnel syndrome.

Diseases. Metabolic diseases (such as diabetes, thyroid disease, and amyloidosis) and autoimmune diseases (such as rheumatoid arthritis, lupus, and connective tissue disorders) have been linked to a higher risk of developing carpal tunnel syndrome.

Previous bone dislocation or fracture. These injuries may cause bones to protrude into the carpal tunnel, narrowing it.

Hormone status. Approximately 20% of pregnant women develop carpal tunnel syndrome during their last trimester, most likely because of fluid retention caused by hormones. Symptoms usually disappear gradually after the baby is delivered. Having your ovaries removed (surgical menopause) also appears to increase the risk.

Body weight. Being overweight or obese appears to raise the risk—perhaps as much as twofold.

Wrist position. Keeping your wrists bent while sleeping, reading, or driving may contribute to carpal tunnel syndrome.

Occupation. Multiple excellent studies dispel the notion that carpal tunnel syndrome stems from computer use or repetitive motion. Occupations that have been linked to carpal tunnel syndrome involve the use of vibrating power tools, especially in a cold environment. For example, meatpackers who use chain saws in a refrigeration locker are prone to the problem, as are workers in the logging industry. However, these cases are most often seen in younger men. There also appears to be an association in these occupational groups between carpal tunnel syndrome and workplace-related Raynaud's syndrome, which is also linked to the use of vibrating tools.

Diagnosing carpal tunnel syndrome

Your doctor will ask you to describe your symptoms and to recall when and how often they occur and how severe they are. He or she will examine your hands, arms, shoulders, and neck to determine whether the complaints might be related to daily activities and rule out other conditions that might mimic carpal tunnel syndrome. Routine laboratory tests, including x-rays and blood tests, which can reveal diabetes, arthritis, and fractures, may also be done. The doctor will examine your wrists and hands for signs of tenderness and swelling and test the sensation in each finger. He or she will also assess the muscles at the base of your hand to see if they show signs of weakness.

In addition, doctors use specific tests to try to elicit the symptoms of carpal tunnel syndrome. In the Tinel test, the doctor taps or presses on the median nerve. If that causes a shock or tingling in the fingers, the test is positive, meaning you may have carpal tunnel syndrome. The Phalen, or wrist-flexion, test involves holding the elbows straight and flexing the hands and wrists. This test is positive if your fingers tingle or feel numb within one minute. The Durkan, or carpal compression, test involves putting pressure directly over the nerve and is positive if the fingers feel numb or tingly within 30 seconds.

Symptoms of carpal tunnel syndrome

- ✔ Pain, weakness, tingling, and numbness in the thumb, index and middle fingers, and half of the ring finger, especially at night
- ✔ Difficulty making a fist, grasping small objects, or doing other manual tasks

You may need additional tests to confirm the diagnosis. One is a nerve conduction test (also called a nerve conduction velocity or NCV test), which uses a machine that administers weak electric shocks via small electrodes placed on the hands and wrist. The electrodes measure how quickly the nerves are able to transmit impulses. There is a very brief painful sensation during each shock. In another test known as electromyography (EMG), the clinician inserts into the muscle a fine needle that measures electrical activity, which reveals the severity of any damage to the median nerve.

More recently, ultrasound has been used to confirm the diagnosis. This is a noninvasive procedure that causes no pain. Ultrasound can show enlargement of the nerve at the entrance to the carpal tunnel, a common characteristic of carpal tunnel syndrome. It cannot assess other nerve abnormalities, such as spine issues in the neck region or damage to multiple nerves, in the same way EMG can. Your physician can decide which test is better for you.

To determine how compressed your median nerve may be, and whether it is interfering with sensation in your hand enough to place you at risk for burning or cutting yourself, a clinician may measure your ability to feel the pressure from being poked with a strand of nylon (called the Semmes-Weinstein monofilament test). In addition, he or she may test the shortest distance you can detect between two points on your hand being touched (called the Weber 2-point discrimination test).

Treating carpal tunnel syndrome

If you have underlying health problems that may be contributing to carpal tunnel syndrome, such as diabetes or arthritis, they should be diagnosed and treated for your overall health.

Self-help. It's important to rest the affected hand for at least two weeks, avoiding any activities that make your symptoms worse. Because bending the wrist down or up can make symptoms worse, it can help to wear a splint that keeps your wrist in a neutral position (see photo, above right). Many people find that wearing a splint at night is an effective treatment, especially if they tend to bend their wrists during sleep. If your symptoms are new, you may only need to wear the splint at night until they resolve. For chronic carpal tunnel syndrome, it may be a long-term way to manage your symptoms without surgery.

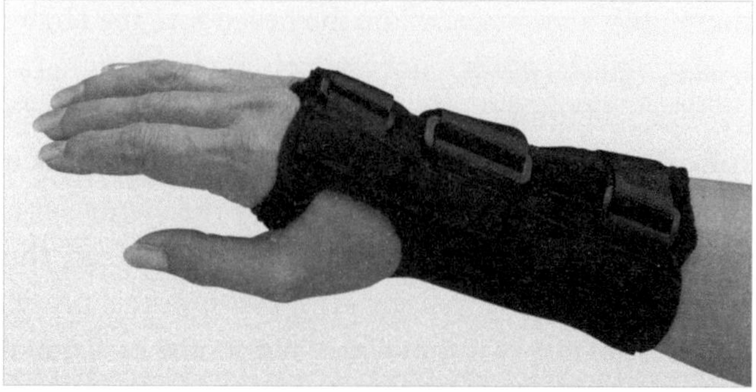

Courtesy North Coast Medical

This is one of many brands of prefabricated wrist splints for carpal tunnel syndrome. It keeps the wrist in a neutral position, while allowing the fingers and thumb to move freely. Consult a hand therapist to help you choose and adjust your splint. Wear it only at night. This splint can also be used for a ganglion cyst.

Medications. There's no evidence that ordinary NSAIDs such as aspirin, ibuprofen (Advil), and naproxen (Aleve) are effective for treating carpal tunnel syndrome. The same goes for the COX-2 inhibitor celecoxib (Celebrex). On rare occasions, some doctors prescribe corticosteroid pills for the short-term relief of symptoms (perhaps while awaiting surgery), but these shouldn't be taken for more than one or two weeks. People with diabetes may experience elevated blood sugar levels and should consult with their diabetes specialist before taking corticosteroids.

Hand therapy. Hand therapy for carpal tunnel syndrome focuses on decreasing the pressure on the median nerve in the carpal tunnel and increasing circulation to the area. It is most effective if it takes place before symptoms are severe. The therapist will work with you on ways to treat the problem, such as wearing a splint at night, adapting tools to lessen vibrations, pacing or rotating tasks at work, and learning how to keep the wrist in a neutral position during activities. Gentle hand exercises may or may not be prescribed, depending on your situation. Avoid squeezing a therapy ball or sponge, as it will not help with carpal tunnel syndrome and may only worsen the condition. Specific tendon-gliding exercises may be suggested to relieve pain and tingling by improving the way your tendons move through the carpal tunnel, but these can irritate the nerve and need to be done cautiously and under the guidance of a therapist. If you have constant numbness or atrophy of your thumb muscles, you should be evaluated by a hand surgeon.

Injections. Corticosteroid injections into the carpal tunnel may relieve symptoms, especially in younger people who have had symptoms only for a short time. Studies on the long-term benefits of steroid injections have had mixed results; for around half of people, the symptoms return within six months.

Surgery. Many people improve with one or more of the above treatments. However, if you have persistent numbness and pain, you feel clumsy and are constantly dropping things, or you are losing muscle mass in your thumb, surgery may be the right choice for you. Usually, it is recommended only if your symptoms last longer than six months. However, people older than 65 may benefit from earlier treatment, because their symptoms tend to progress more quickly and be more debilitating.

The goal of surgery is to create more space in the tunnel by releasing the transverse carpal ligament, which relieves pressure on the median nerve (see "Carrie's story," below). Many procedures are done using local anesthesia and don't require an overnight hospital stay. There are two basic approaches to carpal tunnel release—open and endoscopic—plus a variation on the first called small palmar incision surgery, or the mini-open (so called because it is much smaller than a traditional open release).

- **Mini-open or small palmar incision surgery,** currently the most commonly performed technique, involves an incision less than an inch long in the base of the palm. The idea is to keep the incision small enough to avoid a long recovery, but large enough that the surgeon can see clearly and avoid injuring any nearby tissues. Recovery time is simi-

CARRIE'S STORY:
Surgery to treat carpal tunnel syndrome

When Carrie, a 46-year-old physician assistant, could no longer reliably hold medical instruments, she talked to a surgeon about her carpal tunnel syndrome. This is her story:

I first had problems with numbness and tingling in my hands during the second half of both of my pregnancies as my body started retaining water. Both times it improved within a few weeks of delivery, but then it returned and worsened over the next few years. I'm a physician assistant, so I need to be able to hold instruments and do detailed work with my hands. My thumb, pointer, middle, and ring fingers would get uncomfortably numb, and eventually I couldn't feel and grip things well enough to be sure I wouldn't drop something.

I had surgery on my right hand in 2017. By that time, wearing splints at night didn't alleviate problems during the day, and I had to avoid routine activities that would aggravate the symptoms, like blow-drying my hair, opening jars, sewing, and drawing. I probably waited too long to have surgery, but it was a success.

In 2021, my left-hand numbness got worse and nighttime splints no longer helped, so I decided that enough was enough. It's always a hard decision to have surgery on your hands when your work and your hobbies all involve your hands, but I was told that if I took care of it before there was permanent nerve damage from the ongoing

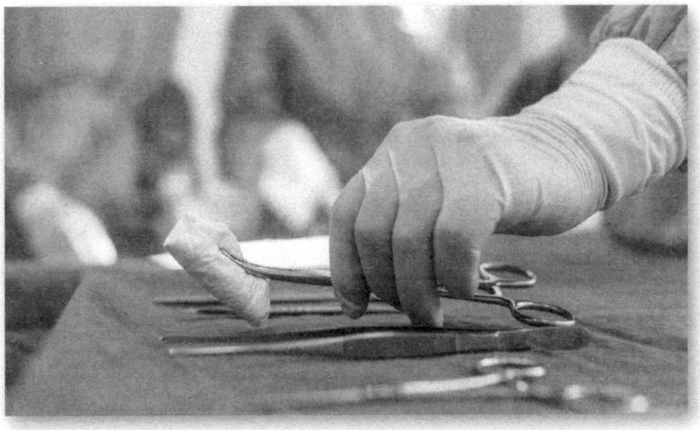

compression, there was a chance I could go back to using my hands normally.

What's great is that it's a quick day procedure. The first time, I had to have stitches removed, but this time they used dissolvable stitches and glue—no cast or splint, not even a bandage. I iced and propped my hand up on pillows until the swelling went down. At my two-week check, I had a full range of motion so I didn't need hand therapy; the only restriction was to not lift anything heavier than 5 pounds for six weeks and not to do anything that put my full weight on my hands—like a plank exercise—for a few months.

Six weeks after surgery, I'm back at work, with a few restrictions. I don't wake up with numbness, and I can use the keyboard, hold my phone, grip the steering wheel, and get back to my crafts. The only thing I'm still struggling with a little is getting back my grip strength so I don't need help opening jars.

lar to that for the endoscopic procedure described below.

- **Traditional, or open, surgery** consists of making an incision up to two inches long in the hand and wrist, often crossing the wrist crease, to alleviate pressure within the carpal tunnel. This technique has the advantage of allowing the surgeon to see the anatomy of your wrist clearly, which lessens the risk for injury to nearby nerves and other vital structures. But with open surgery the scar is more likely to be tender, and the recovery period longer, compared with mini-open surgery.
- **Endoscopic surgery** involves making one or two smaller (half-inch) incisions in the wrist and palm. The surgeon inserts a tiny camera attached to a slender tube (endoscope) through one incision, views the tissue on a screen, and uses tiny surgical tools, also inserted through an incision, to cut the carpal ligament. The smaller incisions minimize scarring and speed recovery compared with the open and mini-open procedures. However, endoscopic surgery has a higher risk for complications, such as damage to the median or ulnar nerve.

Most surgeons prefer one technique over the others. Many feel that the risks involved with the endoscopic technique—although extremely low—aren't worth the potential improvement in recovery time.

Success rates for these surgeries are high, with 80% to 90% of people reporting relief of daytime and nighttime symptoms after six weeks. But people vary significantly in how quickly they recover. You can expect to resume your strength more gradually, and it may take a year or two before you feel you're back to normal.

Researchers at Harvard's Brigham and Women's Hospital conducted a 13-year follow-up of people who received the mini-open surgery. Eighty-eight percent of the 113 people who responded to the survey said they were completely or very satisfied with the results. Asked about their current symptoms, 87% reported good results, and fewer than 2% needed repeat carpal tunnel surgery. In a larger retrospective study of complications in 904 patients treated at Brigham and Women's Hospital, 1.2% developed a complication, with no cases of major injury to nerves or blood vessels.

Hand dystonias: Writer's cramp and musician's cramp

© bubaone | Getty Images

Writer's cramp, a rare condition characterized by an abnormally tight grip on the pen and awkward hand, wrist, and elbow positions, is sometimes mistaken for repetitive strain injury. But it's actually a form of dystonia, a neurological problem that results in sudden, involuntary muscle contractions.

So-called focal dystonias are localized to a particular part of the body and can affect muscles in such places as the neck, eyelids, and vocal cords. They usually occur only in people who assume abnormal positions for long time periods, and only when they perform specific tasks. In adults, focal dystonia of the hand is perhaps the best known, although it accounts for only a tiny fraction of hand conditions. Writer's cramp (also called musician's cramp) is a spasmodic contraction of the muscles of the hand and forearm. The fingers may suddenly freeze up, dramatically affecting the ability to write or play an instrument. Some golfers experience hand dystonias while putting, a phenomenon that's been nicknamed "the yips."

These uncommon afflictions are thought to stem from abnormal functioning of a deep brain structure called the basal ganglia, which initiates and controls the body's movements. Researchers believe that an imbalance of the neurotransmitter dopamine may underlie some forms of dystonia. As with many medical conditions, anxiety and stress—common among professional musicians and athletes during performances—seem to make the problem worse.

Several medications used to treat Parkinson's disease, including trihexyphenidyl (Artane) and benztropine (Cogentin), have been tested for writer's cramp, but the side effects usually aren't worth the small benefit. Another treatment that's gained interest is the injection of botulinum toxin type A (Botox), a substance best known for its cosmetic use to erase wrinkles in the face. A study in the journal *Neurology* found that 69% of musicians with musician's cramp were helped by the injections. A review of studies on the use of botulinum toxin injections to treat writer's cramp found that 50% to 70% of patients were helped. Muscle weakness was a common side effect, both in those who got relief from their cramps and in those who did not.

Repetitive strain injury

Certain work-related medical conditions that affect the body's upper extremities and the neck fall under the broad category of musculoskeletal disorders and are variously known as repetitive strain injury, repetitive stress injury, cumulative trauma disorder, or overuse syndrome. These conditions are more common in manufacturing, food processing, and other industries where workers carry out repetitive motions.

Prolonged computer keyboard use may also put you at risk for repetitive strain injury. Excessive typing and contracting the forearm and wrist muscles for long periods of time can lead to pain, tenderness, and tingling in the arms and fingers, although there is not a clear source of injury to the muscles and joints responsible for the discomfort. Other factors that can contribute to problems include incorrect positioning of the keyboard and computer mouse, use of a laptop rather than a desktop computer, and sustained use of a computer mouse. Carpal tunnel syndrome is sometimes misclassified as a repetitive strain injury. Although some symptoms can be the same, there are important differences; carpal tunnel syndrome is specifically caused by pressure on the median nerve in your wrist, while repetitive strain injury can involve nerves, muscles, and tendons in the wrist, elbow, and shoulder. Carpal tunnel syndrome is not caused by repetitive motion.

Help for computer-related hand problems

If you work in an office, it's a good idea to have an ergonomic evaluation of your workspace to avoid habits that may put you at risk for a variety of musculoskeletal disorders. If that's not possible—for example, because you're working from a home office—the following tips may help:

- Keep your wrists in a neutral position, not flexed downward or extended upward, when using your computer. To check, place your forearm and hand, palm facing down, on a flat, hard surface with your wrist straight. Put a Band-Aid lengthwise over the top of your wrist, and then move to your keyboard and type. If the Band-Aid stretches or goes slack, your wrists aren't in a neutral position.
- Get up from your desk and stretch at least once every hour. In between, take shorter breaks from continuous typing (every 10 or 20 minutes) to rest your hands, palms up, on your lap or on a wrist rest. You can set a smartphone reminder or install software on your computer that reminds you to take rest breaks and restricts your daily time on the computer.
- Avoid the use of a laptop computer. A desktop model with a detached keyboard is a better solution, as it puts less strain on the hands and wrists. Also, be skeptical about keyboard configurations (such as split keyboards) or mouse designs claiming to be ergonomic. It will take many years of study to learn whether such changes translate into fewer work-related upper-extremity musculoskeletal disorders.
- Do not use splints or anti-inflammatory medicine to mask your symptoms so you can type more, because this may make the problem worse. Instead, use splints at night when you are resting.
- See a hand therapist to learn exercises and stretching techniques to ease discomfort.

Ergonomics specialists who design strategies to improve the fit between workers and their jobs suggest the following arrangement for computer workstations:

- Keep documents, telephone, keyboard, mouse, and supplies within easy horizontal reach—not more than 16 to 18 inches away.
- Place the computer monitor directly in front of you, at arm's length, with the top line of the screen at or slightly below eye level (possibly lower for someone with bifocals or trifocals).
- Set your keyboard on an adjustable tray so that your forearms are parallel to the floor, wrists are straight and in line with your forearms, and elbows are relaxed and bent at a 90° angle at your waist.
- Keep your mouse close to the keyboard at the same height so that your elbow stays by your side.
- Consider using voice-activated computer programs.
- Use an adjustable chair, with a rounded front edge and good lower- and upper-back support, positioned so that your knees are slightly lower than your hips, and your feet rest firmly on the floor (or on a footrest).

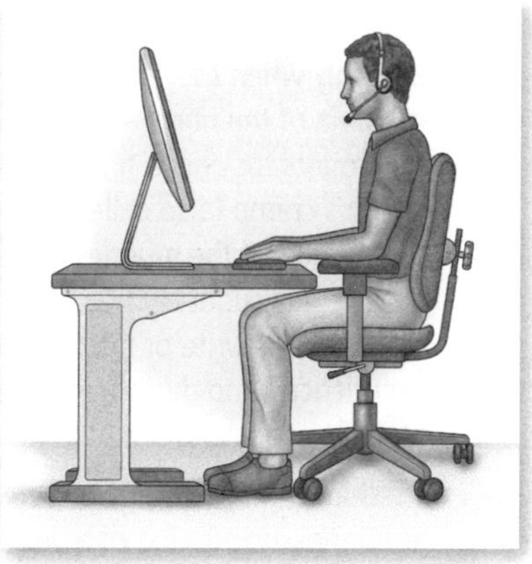

Treating repetitive strain injury

Treating repetitive strain injury largely involves easing the tension in your hands, wrists, and forearms. For heavy computer users, the first step is creating a workspace that minimizes awkward postures and arm movements (see "Help for computer-related hand problems," page 35). If better positioning and self-care don't help, you may need to see a therapist. Therapy may include ice, heat, ultrasound, massage, or various exercises and stretches for the hand.

Cubital tunnel syndrome

The ulnar nerve connects the spinal cord to the muscles of the forearm and hand, as well as the skin on the small-finger side of the hand. When you hit your "funny bone"—the bony bump on the inner side of your elbow, or medial epicondyle—the sensation you feel isn't from the bone itself but from the ulnar nerve, which passes just behind it at the elbow. At that spot, where the bones of the upper and lower arm meet, the nerve is protected only by skin and fat. Hitting that

JONATHAN'S STORY:

Coping with multiple performance-related injuries

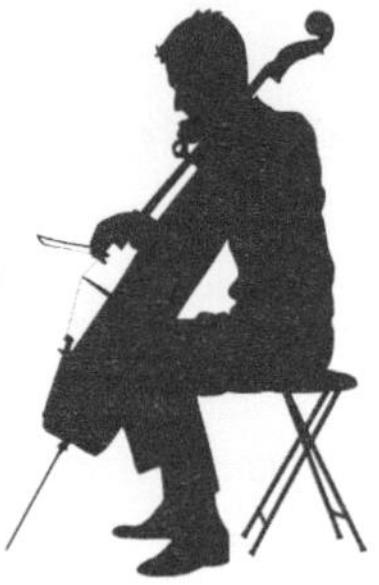

© aarrows | Getty Images

As a professional cellist, Jonathan, then 30 years old, practiced for three to four hours at a stretch and traveled the world for performances, teaching assignments, and auditions. Then, during his third audition in 10 days, his ring finger gave out when he pressed it on a string, and he left the stage fearing that his career was about to be lost. This is Jonathan's story:

My primary care doctor thought my symptoms sounded like tendinitis, and he referred me to a physical therapist who treated me for compression of the nerves between my collarbone and ribs. But after five months of not playing my instrument and of wearing generic splints I had bought off the Internet, I wasn't any better. That time was wasted because I didn't have the right diagnosis! When I finally saw a neurologist in the Performing Arts Clinical Program at the Brigham and Women's Hospital, I was found to have many problems, but not the one I had been treated for. My ulnar nerves were entrapped in both arms—a problem known medically as cubital tunnel syndrome. This created the weakness in my fourth and fifth fingers (the third and fourth in cello fingering). I also had tendinitis in my forearms, trigger fingers, Raynaud's syndrome, and "zingers" from inflamed nerve endings in my left fingertips.

The physical and occupational therapists used many modes of treatment, including deep tissue massage, stretching, ultrasound, heat and cold, joint mobilization of my back, kinesiotape on my forearms and upper back, silicone caps to wear over my fingertips to keep from irritating the nerve endings, compression gloves and sleeves, and three splints for sleeping. They gave me exercises for strengthening and stretching and started me on regular aerobic exercise. Every month the neurologist tested the strength in my hands and watched me play for five minutes to see if that provoked the finger weakness from the ulnar neuropathy. There were times when it was really hard to make the five minutes, or even to play at all.

After three months, the neurologist decided I could start practicing in two-minute intervals three times a day. Two months later, I had to play an important concert but needed steroids and anti-inflammatories to make it through, and that set my treatment back a little.

The neurologist and the occupational therapist recommended several changes to the setup of my instrument, including a lighter bow and cello case, a lower bridge so I don't have to press the strings as hard, a longer nut so the half-steps are closer together, putting New-Skin on my fingertips since I don't have thick calluses to protect the nerve endings, and switching to posture pegs—tuning pegs that don't stick out near my ear so I can play with better posture and easier movement. The posture peg change was an immediate slice of heaven.

There were also a million big surprises about things I was doing wrong in everyday life. Now I've learned to sleep without bending my arms, use earbuds to talk on the phone, limit my computer typing time, put on gloves before going outside instead of letting the Raynaud's syndrome kick in, wear compression sleeves daily, and wear a hand splint when carrying grocery bags so they don't dig into my palms.

Fifteen months after I started being treated at the performing arts clinic, I would say I'm symptom-free, but to stay that way I don't practice more than 30 minutes at a stretch. I also get weekly massages, take Pilates lessons a few times a week to work on symmetry in my body, and use all kinds of tools, such as moist heating pads, to stay healthy. Looking back, except for being told to play in a "relaxed" way, I never got advice about how to prevent or deal with injuries. We musicians need to be more like dancers and sportspeople in how we train and play and use our bodies.

spot traumatizes the nerve, triggering a short-lived shock and tingling sensation, which can radiate down to the ring and little fingers.

The ulnar nerve can also become compressed or irritated at the elbow—a condition known as cubital tunnel syndrome. When you bend your elbow more than 90°, you stretch the ulnar nerve and often pinch the nerve beneath tight overlying tissues. Tasks that require you to bend and straighten your elbow repeatedly can irritate and inflame the nerve. In some people, the nerve shifts and snaps out of its bony groove over the medial epicondyle at the elbow. Leaning or resting on the elbow for long periods (while driving, for instance) can also put pressure on the nerve, as can holding a phone to your ear. The condition is sometimes seen in professional musicians such as pianists and violinists (see "Jonathan's story," page 36). As with carpal tunnel syndrome, your sleep position may aggravate the problem. People with cubital tunnel syndrome often sleep with bent elbows, sometimes with their hands above the head. Injuries are another potential cause of damage to this nerve.

Symptoms of cubital tunnel syndrome include numbness or tingling in the ring and little fingers. Your hands may become weak and clumsy, and you may have trouble straightening your fingers. Touching the elbow may cause a sudden, sharp pain.

Symptoms of cubital tunnel syndrome

- ✔ Numbness, tingling, or pain in the ring and little fingers
- ✔ Weakness or clumsiness of the hand
- ✔ Sharp, sudden pain on the inner elbow when touched

To diagnose cubital tunnel syndrome, the doctor will examine your hand and elbow and ask about your daily work and habits. You may also undergo an x-ray, an NCV test, ultrasound, or electromyography.

Treating cubital tunnel syndrome

Most treatment for cubital tunnel syndrome centers on changing the actions that may have triggered the problem. For instance, switching to a headset-style phone and removing armrests from your office chair may help. Avoid leaning on your elbow, keeping your elbow flexed more than 90°, and doing repetitive actions that require you to bend and straighten your elbow. If you sleep on your back with your arms bent over your head, try sleeping on your side with a pillow supporting the entire length of the arm. A hand therapist may recommend that you wear a soft splint at night to keep your elbow straight and alleviate pressure on the nerve while you are sleeping (see photo at right). A soft kneepad or elbow pad from a sports store, worn on the inside of the elbow, may also help. Your therapist will be able to make a recommendation or fabricate an effective splint. Also, medications to reduce swelling may help (see Table 2, page 9).

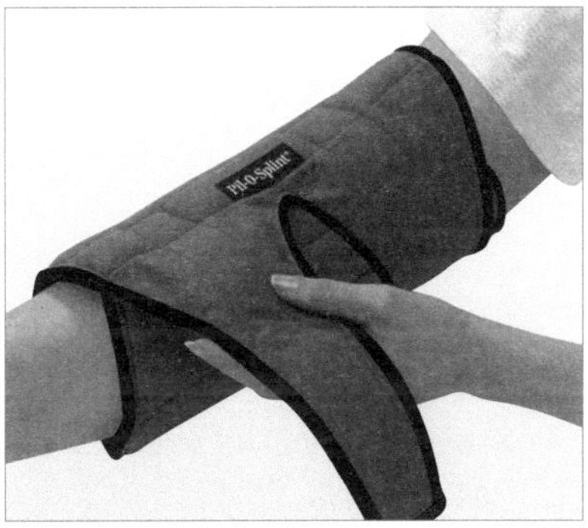

Soft splint for nighttime use

Courtesy Performance Health

About four out of five people improve with these conservative approaches. If you don't, your doctor may suggest surgery, such as ulnar nerve release.

Traumatic hand and wrist injuries

Considering how often you use your hands, it's no surprise that these vital structures are frequently injured. One-third of all injuries seen in emergency rooms involve the hands and arms.

Falls are one of the most frequent causes of these injuries. Many sports, from baseball to rollerblading, also put the hands in harm's way. In fact, about a quarter of all athletic injuries affect the hands and wrists. People in motor vehicle accidents often sustain hand and wrist injuries. Power tools or equipment—especially lawn mowers and snow blowers—are yet another source of danger to the digits.

Most hand injuries are sprains or fractures, both of which can cause swelling, pain, and stiffness and may limit your hand mobility.

A sprain occurs when you stretch or partially tear a ligament, usually from a fall, a sudden twist, or an impact that jolts a joint out of its normal position. Contrary to popular belief, a severe sprain can be as debilitating and painful as a broken bone, and it may take longer to heal because ligaments heal more slowly than bones. The tendons of the hand are also vulnerable to injury, most often from a cut or a jammed finger, which can tear the tendons away from the bones.

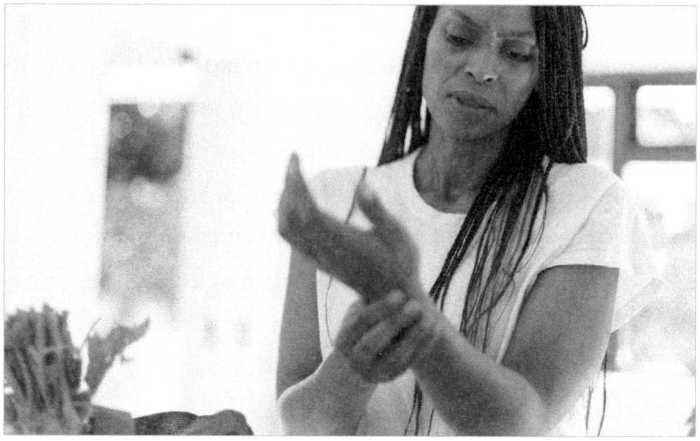

Landing on your palm during a fall—which doctors call a "fall on outstretched hand," or FOOSH—can cause a wrist sprain or even a scaphoid bone fracture in the wrist that feels like a sprain.

Should I see a doctor?

Some sprains are minor and will get better with home treatment that includes RICE (see "First aid: The RICE regimen," page 39), together with pain medications, such as NSAIDs. But other sprains should be evaluated by a health care professional in case you need additional treatment or x-rays to rule out a broken bone. You should consult a clinician if any of the following occurs:

- You have severe pain and cannot put any pressure on the injured joint.
- The injured area looks crooked or has lumps and bumps (other than swelling) that you do not see on the uninjured joint.
- You cannot move the injured joint (but note that in some cases you can move the injured area even when you have a fracture).
- You have numbness, coolness, or discoloration in any part of the injured area.
- You see redness or red streaks spreading out from the injury.
- You injure an area that has been injured several times before.
- You are in doubt about the seriousness of the injury or how to care for it.

A fracture occurs when a forceful impact breaks the underlying bone. In a simple (nondisplaced) fracture, the bone pieces remain aligned and stable. In an unstable fracture, the bone is displaced. If the bone shatters, usually from high-energy force, it's known as a comminuted fracture. If a bone fragment has broken through the skin, it is known as an open (compound) fracture. Most bone fractures will heal with time and treatment. However, it may not be possible to save fingers that are severely crushed, mangled, or pierced by a sharp object.

Wrist sprains

Landing on your palm during a fall forces your wrist to bend backward, potentially tearing or stretching the wrist ligaments. In addition to pain and swelling, your

Symptoms of sprain

- ✔ Pain that develops after an injury, especially if the hand or joint twists or bends at an odd angle
- ✔ Swelling and tenderness of the affected area

First aid: The RICE regimen

If you injure your hand in some way, remember the acronym RICE, which stands for rest, ice, compression, and elevation. These four simple steps will help limit pain and additional damage.

Rest the joint for at least 48 hours.

Ice the injury to minimize swelling, but don't apply the ice directly to your skin. Put cubed or crushed ice in a plastic bag, and then wrap the bag in a towel. You can also use an ice pack, a chemical cold pack, or even a bag of frozen vegetables. Keep the ice on the injured area for no longer than 20 minutes at a time.

Compress the injured area with an elastic compression bandage to provide support and reduce swelling. Wrap it so that it's just slightly snug, taking care not to limit blood circulation.

Elevate your hand above the level of your heart, resting it on a pillow or on the arm of a sofa.

wrist may be tender, bruised, or discolored, and you might have felt a popping or tearing sensation inside the wrist. The skin may feel warm.

If you have a moderate sprain, you may need to immobilize your wrist with a splint for anywhere from a few days to several weeks, depending on the severity of the injury.

A severe sprain can tear the ligament away from the bone, possibly taking a small chip of bone along with it. The resulting injury, known as an avulsion fracture, requires medical care, as does any severe sprain. A severe sprain may lead to instability of the small carpal bones in the wrist. Symptoms of a severe sprain may continue for six to 12 weeks.

If you aren't sure about the severity of the injury, see a doctor for an evaulation. Some wrist injuries that feel like sprains may actually be fractures of the scaphoid bone on the thumb side of the wrist (see "Fractures," page 41).

Finger sprains, jams, and dislocations

Fingers are susceptible to injury in athletic activities that involve catching a ball, such as basketball, football, baseball, and softball. The treatment depends on the type of injury and whether the bones have shifted out of place (dislocation). Typically, the finger is jammed, causing swelling followed by subsequent stiffness of the PIP joint. See your doctor to determine whether there is a dislocation or fracture. If no bones are dislocated, treatment may involve both ice and taping the finger to the adjoining finger (buddy taping) or splinting. Usually, you can start using the finger within a week or so, but check with your doctor to be sure.

If the finger appears to be deformed, a dislocation likely has occurred. Dislocation requires reduction (putting the bones back in alignment). A dislocation can be so painful that a person will pull on the finger, with a resultant "snap" as the joint goes back in place. In football, a coach may do this to a player, which is why it's called "coach's finger." The person may need an x-ray to check whether the joint is misaligned or fractured. If so, you will need to see a hand surgeon for further treatment, possibly involving surgery. Jammed fingers, with or without dislocation, can be stiff and painful for many months.

If you take a spill on the slopes with your hand strapped to a ski pole, it's easy to sprain your thumb at the MCP joint—a problem known as skier's or ski-pole thumb. The thumb's main ligament stabilizes the MCP joint. If you tear the ligament, you'll lose some or all of your ability to grasp things between your thumb and index finger. You'll also have bruising, tenderness, and weakness.

A partial tear will need to be immobilized in a cast or splint for about four to six weeks. After that, you can start flexion and extension exercises (see "Exercises for the hands," page 43), but continue wearing the splint for protection until the swelling and tenderness go away. If the ligament is completely torn, you may need surgery, after which you'll likely need to wear a splint or cast while it heals.

Tendon injuries

The flexor tendons, which connect the muscles of the wrist and forearm to the fingertips, also control finger movement. Tears or cuts in these tendons make it painful or impossible to bend your fingers. Cuts are the most common cause of these injuries, which can lead to finger numbness if the nearby nerves are damaged as well. Sports such as football, wrestling, and rugby can also injure these tendons, tearing them from the bone. Since this may happen when one player grabs another player's jersey, catching and pulling a finger, the injury is sometimes known as jersey finger. Repair and rehabilitation of flexor tendons is delicate and precise. The earlier you seek treatment (no more than a week or so after the injury), the greater your chances of a successful repair.

The extensor tendons, which allow you to straighten your fingers and thumb, are just under the skin on the back of your hand and fingers. Because of their location, they can be easily injured, even by a minor cut. If the tip of your finger is hit with enough force that it bends down toward the palm, the tendon can tear (see Figure 13, above). One common cause is a fast-moving baseball, which is why the injury is sometimes called baseball finger. Known medically as mallet finger, this tendon injury can leave the top of your finger near the fingernail red, tender, painful, and slightly swollen. If the tendon is fully detached from the bone, you won't be able to straighten your

Figure 13: Mallet finger (baseball finger)

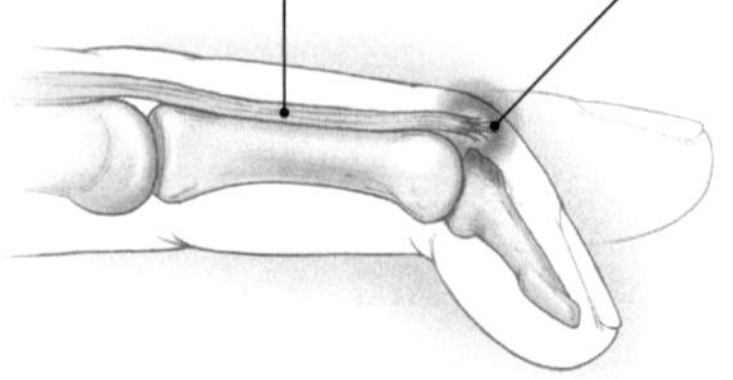

This is a tendon tear caused by a hard blow to the top of the finger. The condition is treated with the use of a splint or small finger cast to immobilize the area for six to eight weeks.

How to prevent falls

1 Make your home environment safer by taking these measures to help fall-proof your house or apartment. (About half of falls happen at home.)

- Remove things you can trip over (such as papers, books, clothes, and shoes) from stairs and places where you walk.
- Remove small throw rugs or use nonskid mats or double-sided tape to keep the rugs from slipping.

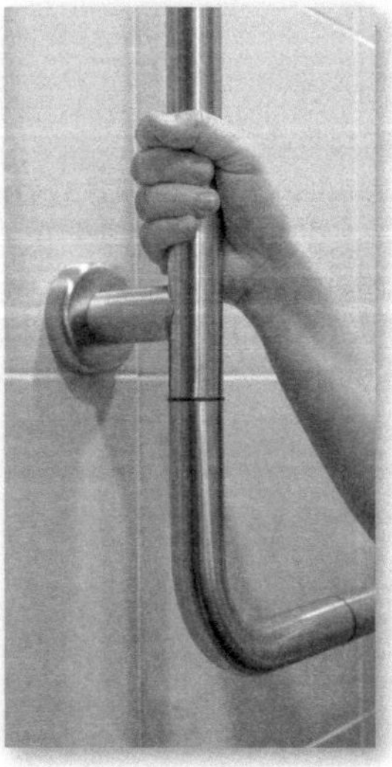

- Keep items you use often in cabinets you can reach easily without using a step stool.
- Install handrails and lights on all staircases.
- Install grab bars next to your toilet and in the tub or shower.
- Use nonslip mats in the bathtub and on shower floors.
- Improve the lighting in your home. As you get older, you need brighter lights to see well. Lamp shades or frosted bulbs can reduce glare.

2 Be sure you are wearing shoes that are stable and fit properly. They should have good support and nonslip soles. Be especially careful when walking outside in snow and ice. Consider getting special cleats that attach to the soles of your shoes to provide extra traction, and, if necessary, get someone to support you as you walk.

3 Don't neglect your exercise. Physical activity helps keep your legs strong and improves your balance and coordination, so you can catch yourself if you stumble.

4 Have your clinician review your medicines, including nonprescription drugs like cold or allergy medications. As you get older, medications may work differently in your body, and certain drugs (and drug combinations) can make you drowsy, potentially leading to a fall.

5 Have your vision checked. If your vision has changed, you may need a new prescription for your glasses. Conditions such as glaucoma or cataracts can also limit vision, increasing your risk for falling.

6 Have your feet checked. Foot problems in seniors increase the risk of falls. Research indicates that among people over age 60, those who experience recurrent falls are more likely to have been bothered by foot pain.

Symptoms of tendon injury

- ✔ Pain and stiffness following an injury
- ✔ Inability to straighten or bend the affected joint

finger, which will hang down in an abnormal position.

While many cut or torn tendons require surgical repair, mallet fingers are most commonly treated without surgery, allowing the tendon to heal on its own, with six to eight weeks of immobilization in a cast or splint. A hand therapist will make sure that your cast or splint keeps your finger fully straight to allow for healing, and can help you to regain mobility after your tendon heals.

Fractures

A broken wrist is the most common fracture among people younger than age 65. The popularity of high-velocity sports that require balance, such as snowboarding and rollerblading, has contributed to an increase in hand and wrist fractures. For older folks, falls can break bones in or near the wrist. Each year, about 29% of adults ages 65 and older fall at least once, according to the CDC. (For tips on fall prevention, see "How to prevent falls," page 40.)

When you fall, your natural reaction is to thrust out your hand to keep your body from hitting the ground too forcefully. On medical charts, doctors refer to the phenomenon with an apt-sounding acronym, FOOSH, which stands for "fall on outstretched hand." What most people refer to as a wrist fracture is actually a fracture of the radius (the main forearm bone) that occurs just above the wrist, in the area called the distal part of the radius. These distal radius fractures are common in adults, especially among middle-aged or older women whose bones have been weakened by osteoporosis. If you break your wrist, many doctors recommend screening for osteoporosis, which can include a bone density scan and blood tests.

A distal radius fracture causes pain and swelling just above the wrist. A doctor may need to reposition the bone and immobilize the wrist with a splint or cast. Sometimes a fracture cannot be adequately realigned by manipulating the bones into place and instead requires surgery. Recovery from treatment for a distal radius fracture may take as long as six to nine months, depending on the severity of the injury. Interestingly, recovery after surgery may be more rapid, sometimes taking as little as three to six months. If you fall on the back of your hand instead of the palm side, the broken bone can shift toward the inside of the wrist. This usually requires surgery to realign the bone fragments.

Another less-common wrist fracture involves the scaphoid bone, also called the navicular bone. One of the eight carpal (wrist) bones that form the carpal tunnel, the scaphoid is a small bone shaped like a cashew on the thumb side of the wrist. Like a dis-

Symptoms of fracture

- ✔ Pain directly over a bone
- ✔ Pain, swelling, and deformity that persist even after following the RICE regimen
- ✔ Inability to move the hand, wrist, or finger

Hand transplantation

First successfully performed in 1998 by a team of surgeons in France, hand transplantation involves the transfer of one or both hands from a deceased human donor to a person who has lost a hand or hands from injury, including severe burns. Unlike a heart or kidney transplant, a hand transplant isn't lifesaving. But for people who have lost one or both hands, the procedure is life-renewing, as everyday activities—from using a fork to touching a loved one—become possible again.

The procedure itself is complicated, involving the transfer of skin, muscle, blood vessels, bones, tendons, and nerves. For this reason, hand transplantation surgery can last anywhere from 12 to 16 hours—about twice as long as a heart transplant. All transplant recipients must take drugs that suppress the immune system for the rest of their lives, so their bodies do not reject the transplanted tissue. Improvements in these medications have helped make hand transplants less risky than in the past.

Worldwide, only a few dozen people have received hand transplants. The procedure is still considered experimental, which means it can only be performed as part of a research study.

Safety tips for using lawn mowers and snow blowers

- Read the instruction manual first.
- Never remove safety devices, including shields or switch guards.
- Keep the machine in good working order.
- Keep children far away from the work area and never allow them to operate these devices.
- Keep your hands and feet clear of all moving parts.
- Never insert hands or feet to remove debris, grass, or snow from these machines. Use a stick or broom handle to remove obstructions.
- Wear protective ear coverings.

- After turning off the machine, wait five seconds for the blades to stop moving.
- Wear protective boots, goggles, gloves, and long pants when mowing a lawn.
- Don't cut wet grass, and be cautious when mowing hills or slopes.
- Keep in mind that the rotating blades are spring-loaded and continue to have energy even when stalled. Therefore, when a locking object is removed, the blade will complete its rotation and potentially cause an amputation.

tal radius fracture, a scaphoid fracture usually results from a FOOSH. It causes pain and tenderness in the wrist and in the area just below the thumb. Sometimes blood from the fractured bone fills the wrist joint, producing visible swelling.

Finger fractures can also occur during falls or other trauma to the hand. Signs of a broken finger include pain when touching the bone, swelling, and difficulty moving the finger. The finger may be displaced or deformed. Some finger fractures only need to be taped, while others need realignment. More complicated fractures may require surgery, during which the doctor may insert pins and screws to hold the broken parts in place.

Finger amputations

Most accidental fingertip amputations occur in young children whose fingers are caught in doors and in men in late middle age who are using power tools. As you'd expect, the middle and index fingers are the most vulnerable. Each year, finger amputations from the use of consumer products send an estimated 23,000 people to hospital emergency departments.

In young children, almost three in four finger amputations result from fingers being jammed or crushed in a door, either in the car or at home. Pinch guards and other safety measures could prevent many of these injuries, experts say. For adults, injuries often occur when a momentary lapse in judgment or failure to follow safety rules, such as wearing proper safety equipment, results in an injury (see "Safety tips for using lawn mowers and snow blowers," above).

If you cut your finger, do the following:

- Elevate the injury and apply ice to reduce bleeding and swelling.
- Cover the finger wound with a dry, sterile dressing.
- Immobilize the affected hand and wrist with a short splint, using any stiff material and tape.

If a finger is completely cut off, take these steps:

- Place the severed finger inside a dry, watertight bag and place the sealed bag in ice water.
- Bring the finger to the emergency room. Depending on the nature and extent of the injury, a surgeon may be able to reattach the finger.

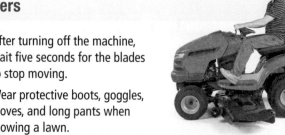

Exercises for the hands

Therapists recommend specific exercises to treat specific conditions. Some exercises help increase your range of motion in a particular joint or lengthen the muscle and its associated tendons (called a muscle-tendon unit) via stretching. These exercises are helpful for osteoarthritis as well as tennis elbow and golfer's elbow—but not when the joints are inflamed or painful. Other exercises strengthen muscles around a joint to generate more power or to give that specific body part greater endurance. These are helpful for resolving tendinitis and nonpainful arthritis conditions.

The following examples describe some commonly recommended exercises for people with hand and wrist problems. But if you have a painful or debilitating hand, wrist, or arm condition, it's best to get specific exercise recommendations from a therapist, rather than exercising on your own. All exercises should be done slowly and deliberately, to avoid pain and injury. If you feel numbness or pain during or after exercising, stop and consult a therapist.

Range-of-motion exercises

Your muscles and tendons move the joints through arcs of motion, as when you bend and straighten your fingers. If your normal range of motion is impaired—if you can't bend your thumb without pain, for example—you may have trouble doing ordinary things like opening a jar. These exercises move your wrist and fingers through their normal ranges of motion and help to lubricate all the hand's tendons by making them glide through their sheaths. Hold each position for five to 10 seconds. Do one set of 10 repetitions, three times a day.

Wrist extension and flexion

- With your arm at your side and elbow bent, position your forearm so your palm faces down.
- Move the hand upward until you feel a gentle stretch.
- Relax the hand back down, bending your wrist until you feel a gentle stretch.

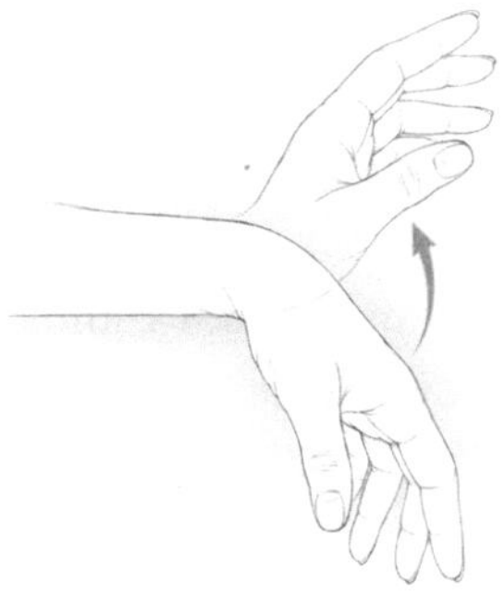

Wrist supination/pronation

- Stand or sit with your arm tucked close to your side with the elbow bent to 90°, palm facing down.
- Rotate your forearm, so that your palm faces up and then down.

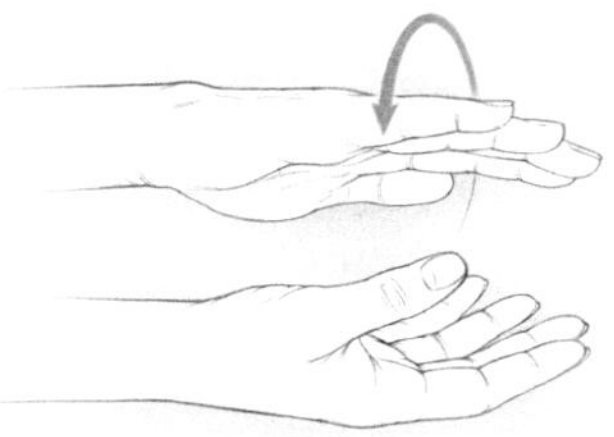

Wrist ulnar/radial deviation

- With your arm at your side and elbow bent, position your hand so your thumb sticks up.
- Wave the hand up and down without moving your forearm.

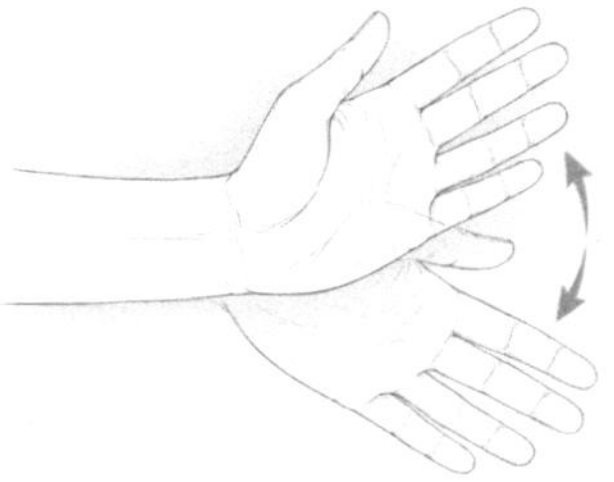

Thumb flexion/extension

- Begin with your thumb positioned straight out to the side.
- Move the thumb across the palm and then back out to the starting position.

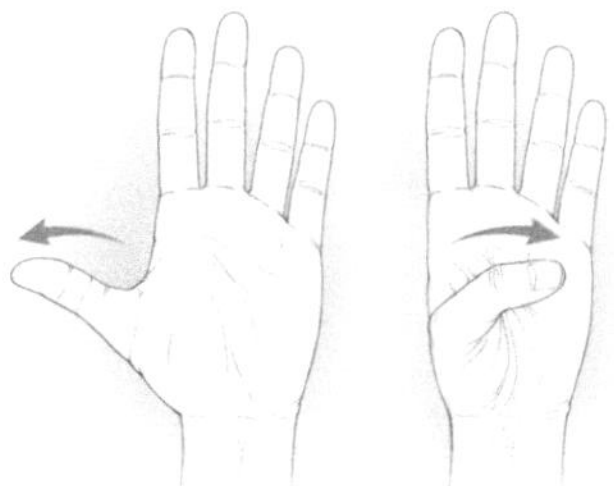

Hand/finger tendon glide

- Start with the fingers extended straight out; keep the wrist in a relaxed, slightly extended position.
- Make a hook fist; return to a straight hand.
- Make a full fist; return to a straight hand.
- Make a straight fist; return to a straight hand.

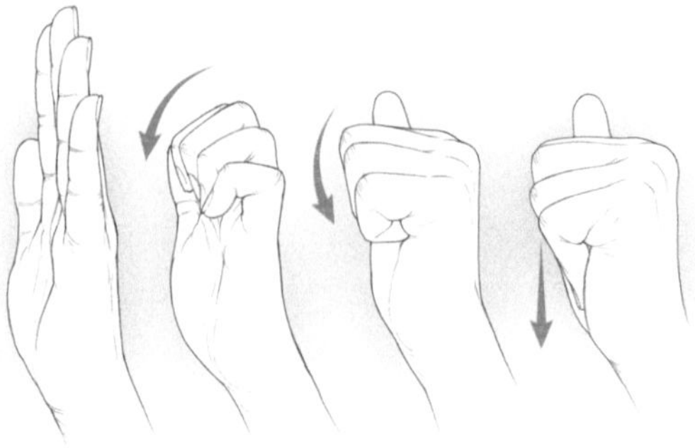

Strengthening exercises

There are two types of exercises for strength.

Using weights. By holding light weights (1 to 3 pounds) during the first three range-of-motion exercises on page 43, you can begin a gentle strengthening program. Increase the weight gradually over time, making sure you can control the motion while holding the weight within a normal (or recommended) range of motion. Begin with one set of 10. If you don't experience any pain over the following 24 hours, gradually build up to doing two to three sets of 10, as tolerated, exercising every other day. Make sure the exercise is not painful or causing any numbness. Do the exercises slowly and deliberately, holding the positions for a count of 5. Be sure to do these only every other day, because your muscles need to rest for 24 to 48 hours.

Using putty. Another set of strengthening exercises for healthy hands involves squeezing a cylinder or ball of putty. Therapy putty, available at medical supply stores and other outlets, is a malleable plastic material used to provide different degrees of resistance for hand exercises to improve grip and pinch strength. Start with the softest putty first and advance only if you can do the exercises without symptoms. You should not feel any pain, numbness, or tingling. You may feel some muscle discomfort after exercise, but it should resolve within 24 hours.

If you have any of the hand conditions described in this report, such as trigger finger, carpal tunnel syndrome, arthritis, or de Quervain's tendinitis, consult a hand therapist for an appropriate exercise prescription. If strengthening exercises are not chosen correctly and performed carefully, they sometimes cause more harm than good.

Putty grip

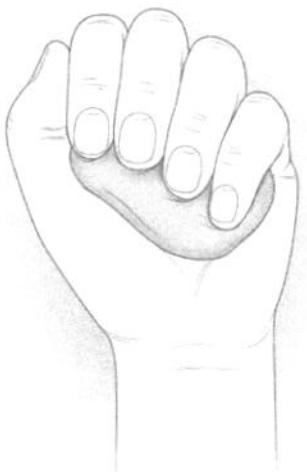

- Roll the putty into a ball.
- Place the putty in your palm.
- Gently squeeze the putty.
- Repeat the sequence 10 times every other day.

Putty key pinch

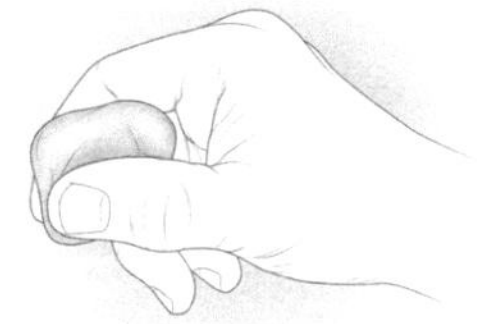

- Roll the putty into a short, fat cylinder.
- Place the putty between your thumb and the side of your index finger.
- Gently squeeze the putty.
- Repeat the sequence 10 times every other day.

Putty three-point pinch

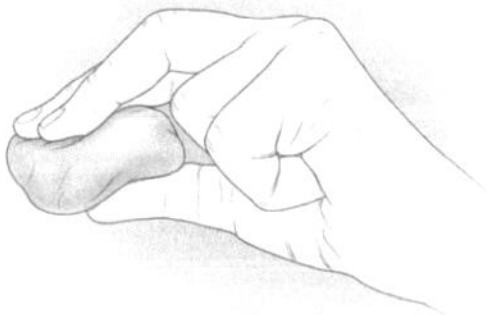

- Roll the putty into a short, fat cylinder.
- Place the putty between the pads of your thumb and your index and middle fingers.
- Gently squeeze the putty between your fingers and thumb.
- Repeat the sequence 10 times every other day.

Stretching exercises

Stretching helps relax stiff, tight muscles and tendons, maximizing the length of the muscle-tendon units in your hands, wrists, and forearms. If you do repetitive tasks, such as typing or gripping gardening tools, you are at particular risk of muscles shortening and becoming tight and painful. Stretching can help counter that problem. These stretches are especially useful for relieving tendinitis and tight forearm muscles, which are common in people who work at computers for long periods of time.

Do these stretches gently, to the point where you feel the stretch but it is not painful. To get the most benefit, do four repetitions of each stretch twice a day, holding the stretch for 30 seconds each time. Rest for 30 seconds between repetitions.

Wrist extensor stretches

- Begin with your arm at your side and elbow bent.
- With the other hand, grasp the thumb side of the hand and bend your wrist downward.
- To increase the stretch, bend your wrist toward your little finger.
- If it doesn't cause pain, repeat the same exercise with the arm out straight in front of you.

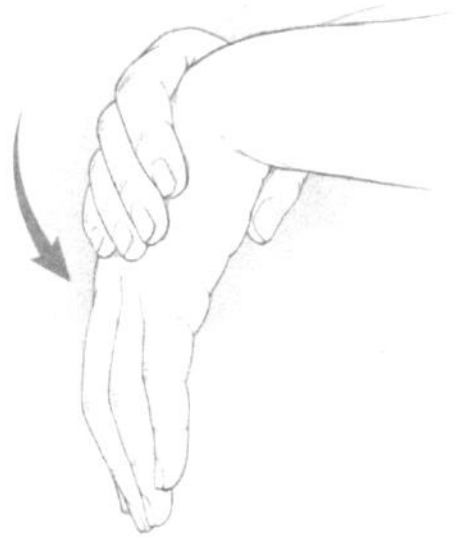

Wrist flexor stretches

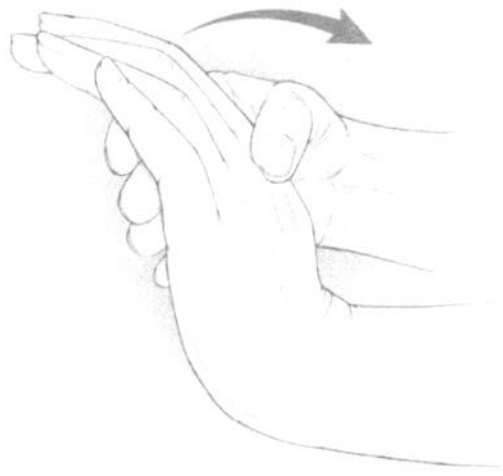

- Begin with a bent elbow.
- Grasp the fingers of that hand with the other.
- Pull the hand back gently.
- If it doesn't cause pain, repeat the same exercise with the arm out straight in front of you.

Resisted isometrics

These exercises keep the joint angle and muscle in the same position as they work against an external force, which provides resistance. Hold the position for 10 seconds, and do one set of 10 repetitions once or twice a day.

Isometric wrist extension

- Hold the affected hand palm down, with the opposite hand on top.
- Try to raise the affected hand, but don't allow either hand to move.

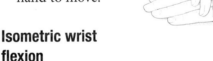

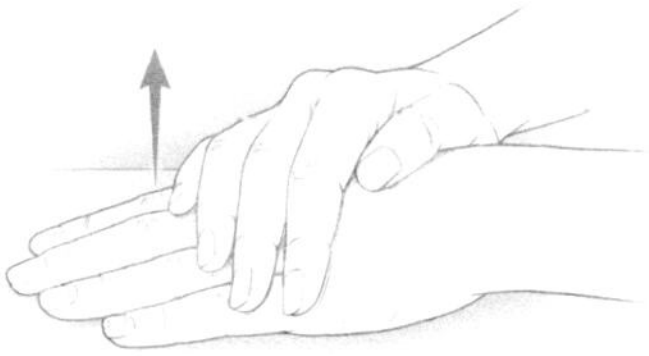

Isometric wrist flexion

- Repeat the same exercise as above, but with the palm facing up.

Dexterity activities

Practicing activities that require quick fine-motor movements of the hands can help counter the loss of dexterity that often occurs with age and in people with nerve compression or osteoarthritis of the hands.

The following provide some good ways to challenge and improve your dexterity:

- Thread buttons or beads onto a thread or ribbon.
- Sort a variety of small objects, such as coins, buttons, or nuts and bolts.
- Shuffle and deal cards.
- Quickly do and undo buttons, snaps, and zippers.
- Work a jigsaw puzzle.
- Rapidly remove and replace small caps and lids from tubes and jars.
- Pick up small objects with your thumb and index finger, then with your thumb and middle finger, thumb and ring finger, and finally the thumb and little finger.

Sensory re-education activities

After surgery involving a nerve, such as surgery to release compression in carpal tunnel syndrome or repair a cut, your doctor may recommend sensory re-education to help you regain the ability to distinguish types and locations of touch on the hands and fingers. In addition to exercises done with a hand therapist, you can work on improving your sensory abilities with these activities:

- Place various coins in your pocket and try to figure out by feel whether you're touching a penny, nickel, dime, or quarter.
- Hide small objects in a bowl filled with rice or dried beans. Reach in and try to identify the objects without using your eyes.
- Attempt to stack objects (such as checkers, coins, or dominoes) with your eyes open, then closed.
- Sort objects (buttons, coins, nuts and bolts) with your eyes open, then closed.

Getting a grip: Handy gadgets and advice

When your hands hurt, everyday tasks like opening a jar or chopping vegetables can be a stressful ordeal. A combination of lifestyle changes and ergonomic tools can help you cope. When you use utensils and tools with enlarged or extended handles, your joints don't have to work as hard and are protected from excessive pressure and strain. Here are some tools and tips that can make your day a little easier; see "Resources," page 50, for suppliers of some of these assistive devices.

In the kitchen

General advice:

- Store frequently used items between shoulder and waist level (for example, in utensil holders on the counter).
- Use a steady footstool to reach higher items.
- Use a rolling cart to move items around the kitchen, and turntables to improve access to items in cupboards.
- When cooking, avoid gripping utensils too tightly.
- Make larger batches of food and freeze extra portions.
- Cook one-pot meals to reduce strain on hands.
- Buy precut produce to reduce peeling and chopping.

Useful gadgets:

- mini chopper
- electric can opener
- jar key opener to release vacuum pressure on a tight lid
- easy-grip five-in-one opener for bottles, jars, cans, and pop-tops
- small nonskid gripper mats to increase traction when opening jars and to place under bowls and other items to prevent slippage
- utensils with built-up padded handles
- loop or spring-loaded scissors (for opening packaged foods and cutting up foods)
- cheese slicer
- bottle brush for washing cups and glasses
- lightweight utensils, pots, and pans
- a rocker knife, which has a curved blade that enables you to cut food on your plate with one hand
- a strap on the refrigerator door (use your arm instead of your hand to pull it open)
- faucet turners at the sink.

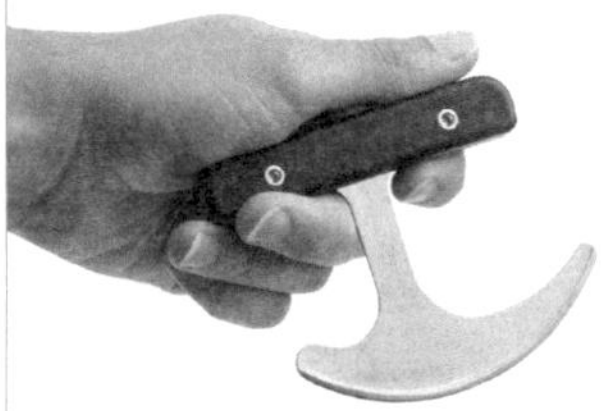

Rocker knife

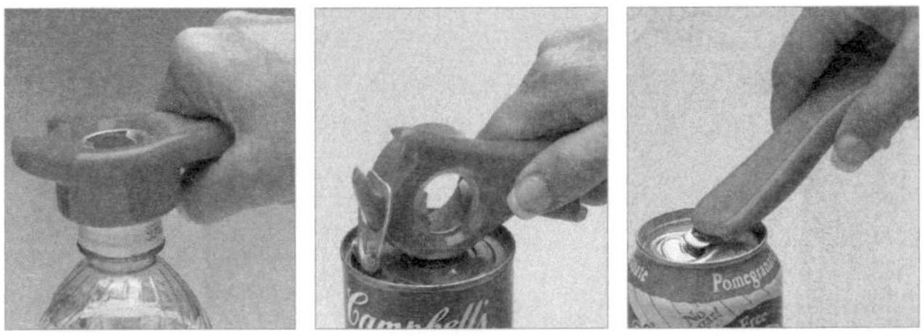

Using the five-in-one device to open a bottle, can, or pop-top.

In the bathroom

General advice:

- Place your most-used items within easy reach.
- If there are no safety concerns, ask your pharmacist to replace childproof caps with tops that are easier to open. If you have dual-purpose tops, flip them to the non-childproof position.
- Fall-proof your bathroom by installing grab bars and textured floor tiles and using nonslip bath mats.

Useful gadgets:

- electric toothbrush
- pump-style toothpaste and soap dispensers
- medicine-bottle opener
- dental floss holder
- electric razor

- soap-on-a-rope or mitts to hold soap in the shower
- brushes or combs with long handles.

In the bedroom

General advice:

- Choose slip-on shoes and loose-fitting garments for easy dressing and undressing.
- Look for clothing with elastic waistbands, large buttons, Velcro fastenings, and zipper pulls.
- Lay your clothes out the night before if you suffer from morning stiffness.
- Fasten your bra in front and turn it around, or choose a front-fastening or pullover style.
- Use a button hook to help button shirts.
- Use a long-handled shoehorn.
- Carry a lightweight purse or briefcase on a strap across your chest or over your shoulder or arm, or consider using a backpack with wide straps or a bag on rolling wheels.
- If you wear jewelry, replace regular clasps with magnetic clasps to make items easier to take on and off.

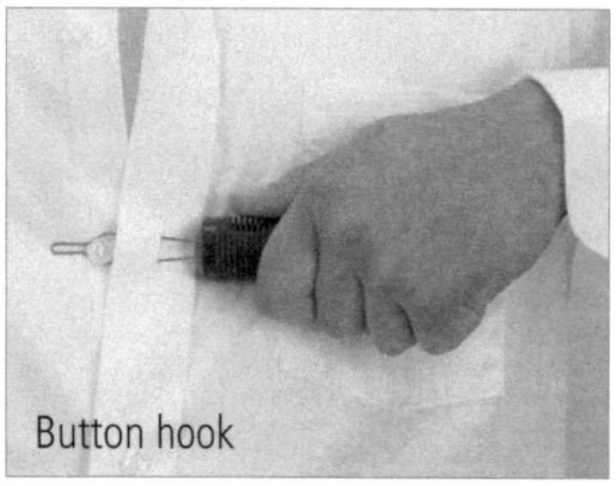
Button hook

Throughout your home and car

General advice:

- When pushing down to stand from a seated position, press with open palms (unless you have wrist problems).
- Strive for good posture; keep your joints in neutral positions.
- Use voice activation on your smartphone whenever you can to minimize repetitive thumb use.
- Don't hold objects (such as a phone) for too long; consider a phone headset.
- Make sure your desk and chair are the correct height for your computer monitor and keyboard.
- When moving heavy items, push rather than pull, and slide rather than lift.
- Spread heavy and light chores throughout the week. Take time to rest!

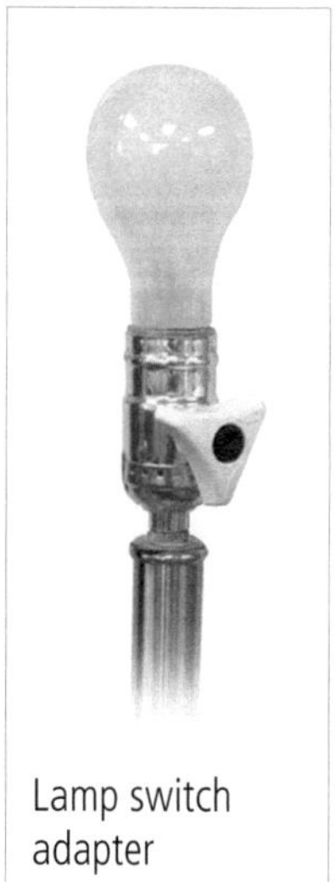
Lamp switch adapter

Useful gadgets:

- key turners
- doorknob extenders
- lamp switch adapters
- lightweight vacuum cleaner
- scissors with padded handles or swivel blades (loop or spring-loaded)
- brooms and mops with built-up, padded handles
- angled shovels
- roller-ball or gel pens and pencils with padded grips
- card holders for playing cards
- book stand
- padding on the steering wheel for a better grip
- extended-handle ice scraper and snow removal brush.

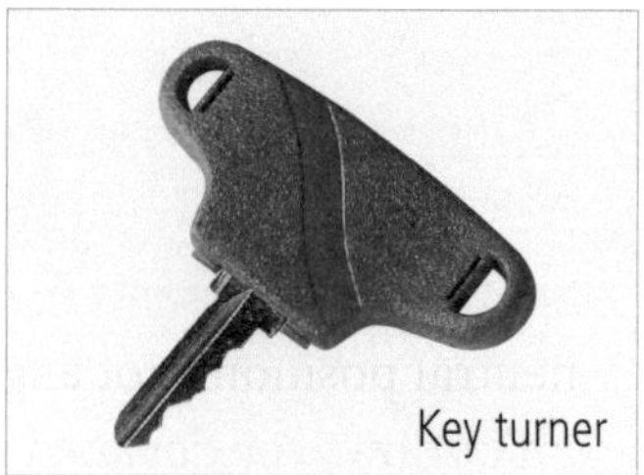
Key turner

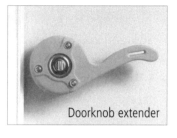

Doorknob extender

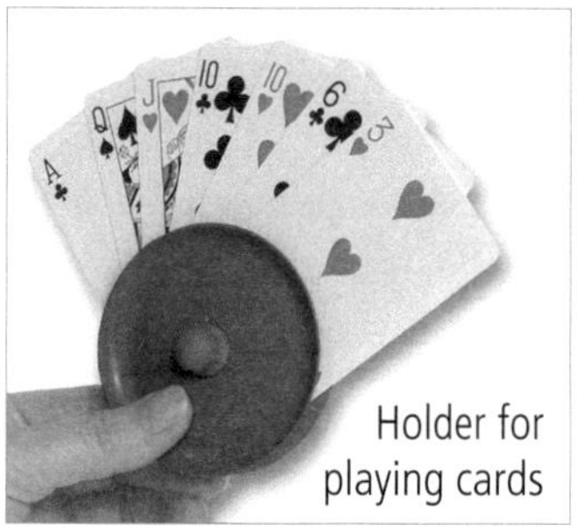
Holder for playing cards

Book stand
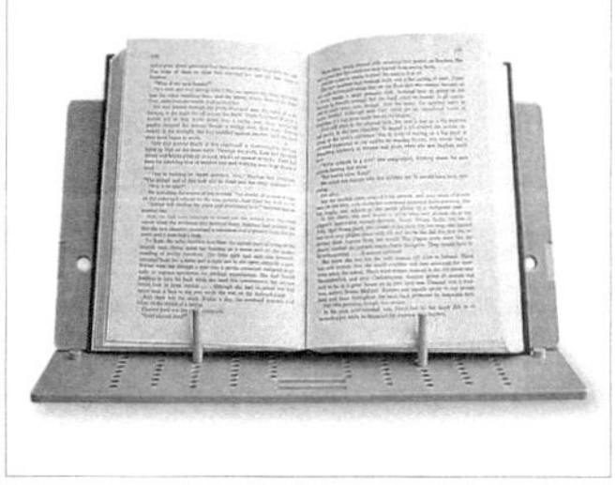

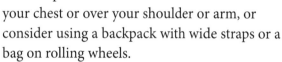

At the grocery store

General advice:

- Buy precut, packaged vegetables and fruits.
- Request paper bags or use recyclable cloth bags, filled with only a few items per bag, and hold them with your forearms facing up, close to your chest.

In the yard and garden

General advice:

- Maintain good posture. Avoid stooping, and try to

Photos courtesy The Wright Stuff

maintain the normal curve of your back. Keep your neck straight, your elbows slightly bent, and your wrists in a neutral position (not angled up or down, or deviated to one side).
- Lift with knees bent, back straight, and palms up.
- Keep your loads light.
- Keep objects close to your body, allowing the larger joints to carry more of the load.
- Work below shoulder level and use both of your arms or hands to accomplish a task whenever possible.
- Hold objects with a light grasp.
- Take frequent breaks, and rotate tasks. Don't do any single activity for an hour without a break.
- Limit overhead activities to 30 minutes, and stop if you notice any numbness. (Numb fingers are not normal and may be a sign of a compressed nerve, possibly in the upper spine or arm. Consult your doctor to pinpoint the cause and find possible solutions.)
- Don't try to do too much in one day; you'll risk pain and disappointment the following days.

Tool tips:

- Choose lightweight gardening tools that have contoured handles to fit your palm. Pick the right tool for the right job, and keep your tools sharp so they'll work more efficiently.
- Tools with built-up, padded handles can lessen joint strain. Tools with short handles give better control, while those with longer handles offer better leverage.
- Wear gloves to protect your hands from chemicals, sharp items, bug bites, and thorns. Gloves also prevent blisters and can decrease potentially nerve-damaging vibrations from power tools. Lightweight cotton or canvas gloves are best for tasks that don't require protection from mud or moisture. Long, rubber, nonslip-grip gloves both protect and add resistance to the hands, but they make fine-motor tasks more difficult. Gloves with special padding and slight compression designed for people with arthritis (such as Womanswork and Manswork) may be more comfortable and improve your grip.
- Ratcheted tools, like a ratcheting pruner, require less effort to use.
- Look for ergonomically designed tools that allow you to garden while standing up.
- Use carts and tool organizers to keep items within easy reach.
- Use a wheelbarrow for heavy loads.
- Use a coiled hose, which is easier to store.

Easy-grip, long-reach fork and cuff

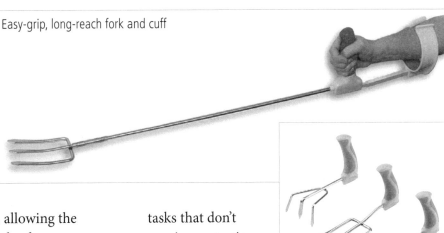

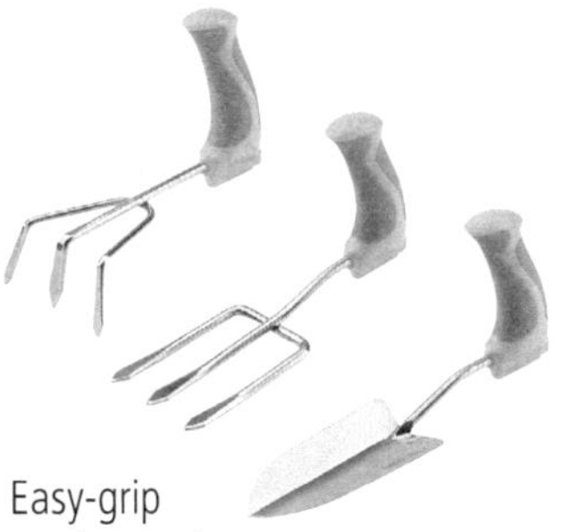

Easy-grip garden tools

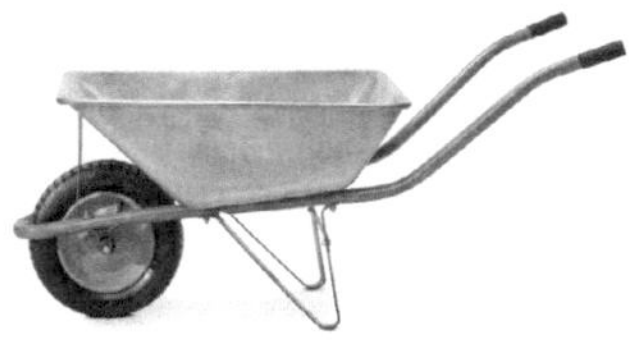

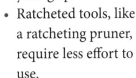

Wheelbarrow for heavy loads

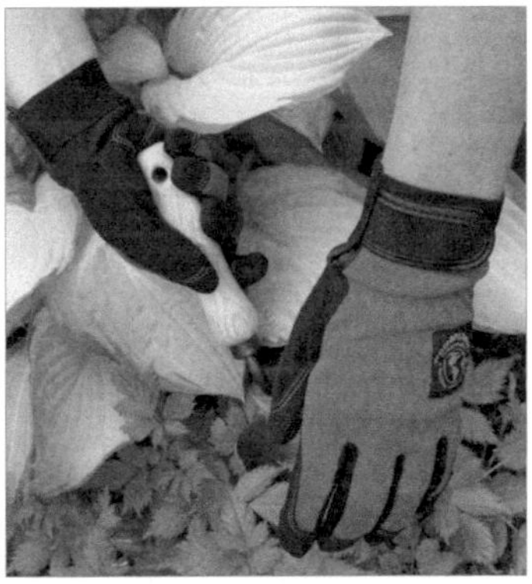

Womanswork digger gloves

Resources

Organizations

American Academy of Orthopaedic Surgeons
9400 W. Higgins Road
Rosemont, IL 60018
847-823-7186
www.aaos.org

This nonprofit organization provides education and services for orthopedic surgeons and other health professionals. The website includes patient information and a doctor referral service.

American College of Rheumatology
2200 Lake Blvd. NE
Atlanta, GA 30319
404-633-3777
www.rheumatology.org

This professional organization of physicians, health professionals, and scientists engages in education, research, and advocacy to improve the care of people with arthritis and other rheumatic and musculoskeletal diseases. The website includes patient fact sheets.

American Occupational Therapy Association
6116 Executive Blvd., Suite 200
North Bethesda, MD 20852
301-652-6611
www.aota.org

This professional organization's website offers information for patients, including free 15-minute podcasts about how occupational therapy can help treat a variety of health conditions.

American Physical Therapy Association
3030 Potomac Ave., Suite 100
Alexandria, VA 22305
800-999-2782 (toll-free)
www.apta.org

This professional organization's website provides a range of information for consumers, including details about therapy for a variety of conditions, an "Ask a PT" feature, and a searchable directory of physical therapists.

American Society for Surgery of the Hand
822 W. Washington Blvd.
Chicago, IL 60607
312-880-1900
www.handcare.org

This professional society provides information for the general public about hand conditions. The website offers a "Find a Surgeon" link.

American Society of Hand Therapists
1120 Route 73, Suite 200
Mount Laurel, NJ 08054
856-380-6856
www.asht.org

This professional organization provides consumer information about common hand conditions and an online searchable index of certified hand therapists.

Arthritis Foundation
1355 Peachtree St. NE, Suite 600
Atlanta, GA 30309
800-283-7800 (toll-free)
www.arthritis.org

This nonprofit foundation sponsors public education programs and continuing education for professionals, raises money for research, and publishes patient information materials. Local chapters can advise about doctors and sponsor activities such as swimming and self-help classes.

Hand Therapy Certification Commission
180 Promenade Circle, Suite 300, #41
Sacramento, CA 95834
800-860-7097 (toll-free) or 916-566-1140
www.htcc.org

This professional organization's website includes a link (under "CHT Directory") that allows you to search for a certified hand therapist in your area.

Performing Arts Medicine Association
P.O. Box 117
Englewood, CO 80151
303-808-5643
www.artsmed.org

This professional organization's website includes a link (under "Referrals") that allows you to search for physicians and other health professionals with a special interest in treating musicians.

Products

BraceLab
2609 Atlantic Ave., Suite 213
Raleigh, NC 27604
888-235-8221 (toll-free)
www.bracelab.com

Braces for the thumb, wrist, and elbow, including the MetaGrip. Have them fitted by a therapist.

Fiskars Brands, Inc.
7800 Discovery Drive
Middleton, WI 53562
608-294-4771
www.fiskars.com

Hand tools for a variety of uses (crafting, gardening, and office work). In any "Products" category, look for the "Easy Action" products, recommended by the Arthritis Foundation.

North Coast Medical, Inc.
780 Jarvis Drive, Suite 100
Morgan Hill, CA 95037
800-821-9319 (toll-free) or 408-766-5000
www.ncmedical.com

Occupational and hand therapy products, rehabilitation products for physical therapy, and ergonomic products for the workplace. Products include dressing aids, household helpers, adaptive eating utensils, exercise equipment, transfer devices, and more.

OXO
1331 S. 7th St., Building 1
Chambersburg, PA 17201
800-545-4411 (toll-free)
www.oxo.com

Consumer products designed to make everyday living easier, including the OXO Good Grips line of tools and housewares.

Performance Health
28100 Torch Parkway, Suite 700
Warrenville, IL 60555
800-323-5547
www.performancehealth.com

Rehabilitation equipment and supplies for the professional and the home.

Silver Ring Splint Company
P.O. Box 2856
Charlottesville, VA 22902
800-311-7028 (toll-free)
www.silverringsplint.com

Splints for a variety of conditions, including boutonniere deformity, trigger finger, and swan-neck deformity.

Harvard Special Health Reports

The following reports from Harvard Medical School offer further detail on topics mentioned in this report. They can be ordered by calling 877-648-9457 (toll-free) or by going to www.health.harvard.edu.

The Joint Pain Relief Workout: Healing exercises for your shoulders, hips, knees, and ankles
Lauren E. Elson, M.D., Medical Editor and Michele Stanten, Fitness Consultant
(Harvard Medical School, 2021)

Designed by a rehabilitation doctor, these workouts are intended to strengthen the muscles that support your joints, increase flexibility in your joints, and improve range of motion. Done regularly, these exercises can ease pain, improve mobility, and help prevent further injury.

Living Well with Osteoarthritis: A guide to keeping your joints healthy
Robert H. Shmerling, M.D., Medical Editor
(Harvard Medical School, 2019)

This report examines the effectiveness, safety, and possible side effects of more than 40 medications used to treat arthritis. It also covers joint replacement surgery, along with physical therapy and complementary procedures. A Special Section covers helpful tools and do-it-yourself solutions.

Rheumatoid Arthritis: How to protect your joints, reduce pain, and improve mobility
Robert H. Shmerling, M.D., Medical Editor
(Harvard Medical School, 2018)

This report covers pain relievers and disease-modifying drugs, along with advances in less-invasive surgery, and practical, no-cost ways to lessen joint stress and pain.

Books

The Hand Owner's Manual: A Hand Surgeon's Thirty-Year Collection of Important Information and Fascinating Facts
Roy A. Meals, M.D.
(Virtualbookworm.com Publishing, 2008)

Practical advice for preventing and treating common hand problems such as pinched nerves, broken bones, and arthritic joints, along with tips for keeping your hands healthy.

One-Handed in a Two-Handed World
Tommye-Karen Mayer
(Prince-Gallison Press, 2013)

A step-by-step guidebook for managing just about everything with the use of one hand, whether your one-handedness is temporary, long-term, or permanent.

Glossary

arthritis: Inflammation of a joint, often with destruction of cartilage.

arthroplasty: Joint replacement surgery.

autoimmune disorder: A condition stemming from an abnormal immune response generated by the body against its own tissues, cells, or molecules.

Bouchard's nodes: Bony nodules that may form in the middle joints of one or more fingers in people with osteoarthritis.

carpal tunnel syndrome: A condition in which the median nerve is compressed as it passes through a narrow space within the wrist, called the carpal tunnel. It is not caused by repetitive motion, though it may be linked to the use of vibrating tools, such as power tools and chain saws.

carpometacarpal (CMC) joint: Joint where a metacarpal bone of the hand and carpal bone of the wrist come together.

cartilage: A type of connective tissue that protects and cushions the ends of bones.

crepitus: Grinding sensation or sound when a joint moves.

cubital tunnel syndrome: A condition in which the ulnar nerve is compressed at the elbow.

de Quervain's tendinitis: Inflammation of tendons at the wrist that move the thumb.

distal interphalangeal (DIP) joint: The last joint before the nail on each finger except the thumb; the most common site for osteoarthritis of the hands.

Dupuytren's disease: A condition that causes abnormal thickening in tissues of the hand that forces one or more fingers to curl toward the palm.

dystonia: Abnormal muscle tone or tension in one or more muscles.

epicondylitis: Degeneration of tendons in the elbow, often the result of overuse.

ergonomics: The science of designing and arranging things people use to enable the safest, most efficient interaction between people and things.

ganglion cyst: A benign, fluid-filled cyst commonly found on the back of the wrist or elsewhere on the hand.

gout: Arthritis caused by uric acid crystals.

Heberden's nodes: Bony and fibrous nodules that may form in the end joints of one or more fingers in people with osteoarthritis.

inflammation: A response to injury or foreign invasion designed to protect the body; the symptoms are heat, redness, swelling, and pain.

ligament: A band of fibrous tissue that connects bones and stabilizes joints.

metacarpophalangeal (MCP) joint: Knuckle joint where a metacarpal bone in the hand and a finger bone come together.

mucous cysts: Small cysts that form between the nail bed and the top joint of the finger, most commonly in people with osteoarthritis.

osteoarthritis: A joint disease common with aging, characterized by progressive deterioration of the cartilage that lines the joints; also called degenerative joint disease.

osteophyte: A bony growth on the edge of a joint, usually caused by osteoarthritis; commonly called a bone spur.

phalanges: The finger bones.

proximal interphalangeal (PIP) joint: The middle joint of the finger.

pseudogout: Arthritis caused by crystals of calcium pyrophosphate dihydrate in the joints; also known as calcium pyrophosphate deposition disease, or CPDD.

psoriasis: A skin disease characterized by thickened patches of inflamed, red skin.

pulleys: Rings of connective tissue that form a tunnel for tendons in the fingers, holding a given tendon to the bone.

Raynaud's syndrome: A condition in which the blood vessels in the fingers and other extremities narrow in response to cold or stress, causing them to turn white or blue.

repetitive strain injury: A type of overuse injury caused by repetitive motions, common in manufacturing, food processing, and jobs involving excessive typing.

rheumatoid arthritis: A chronic autoimmune disorder that causes joints to become painful, inflamed, and sometimes deformed.

scleroderma: A disease of the body's connective tissue that causes the skin to thicken and harden.

sprain: A stretch or incomplete tear in a ligament.

synovectomy: Surgical removal of the synovium.

synovial fluid: A thick fluid that lubricates the joints and tendons.

synovium: A thin membrane that lines joint capsules and produces synovial fluid.

tendon: A tough, fibrous tissue that connects muscle to bone.

tenosynovitis: Swelling and inflammation of the tendon sheath, which decreases the sheath's production of synovial fluid.